Synthesis Lectures on Engineering, Science, and Technology

The focus of this series is general topics, and applications about, and for, engineers and scientists on a wide array of applications, methods and advances. Most titles cover subjects such as professional development, education, and study skills, as well as basic introductory undergraduate material and other topics appropriate for a broader and less technical audience.

Khalid Shaikh • Rohit Thanki • Affaan Shaikh

Artificial Intelligence in Drug Discovery and Development

Springer

Khalid Shaikh
Prognica Labs Tech FZCO
Dubai, Dubai, United Arab Emirates

Rohit Thanki
Wolfsburg, Germany

Affaan Shaikh
Neuratia Labs
Dubai, United Arab Emirates

ISSN 2690-0300 ISSN 2690-0327 (electronic)
Synthesis Lectures on Engineering, Science, and Technology
ISBN 978-3-032-10276-8 ISBN 978-3-032-10277-5 (eBook)
https://doi.org/10.1007/978-3-032-10277-5

This Springer imprint is published by the registered company Springer Nature Switzerland AG
The registered company address is: Gewerbestrasse 11, 6330 Cham, Switzerland

Preface

Artificial intelligence (AI) is rapidly transforming the landscape of drug discovery and development, offering unprecedented opportunities to accelerate biomedical innovation, enhance accuracy, and personalize medical solutions. The core objective of this book is to illuminate the diverse applications of AI across the pharmaceutical spectrum, encompassing target identification, chemical screening, biomarker detection, and clinical trial optimization, while remaining accessible to a broad readership that spans scientists, clinicians, industry leaders, and policy makers.

This book is inspired by the urgent challenges facing the healthcare sector, from rising costs and lengthening development cycles to complex regulatory landscapes and the demand for safer, more effective therapies. By sharing practical insights, current case studies, and critical analysis of evolving technologies, we hope to bridge the gap between technological potential and real-world implementation, empowering stakeholders to leverage AI for impactful drug development. Whether the reader is a pharmaceutical professional seeking to adopt AI tools, a researcher curious about the latest breakthroughs, or an innovator charting the future of healthcare, this book provides a comprehensive road map to the frontier of AI-driven medicine.

Dubai, Dubai, United Arab Emirates — Khalid Shaikh
Wolfsburg, Germany — Rohit Thanki
Dubai, United Arab Emirates — Affaan Shaikh

Acknowledgments

We wish to acknowledge the tireless efforts of mentors, reviewers, and editorial boards whose constructive feedback helped shape the direction and content of this work. Our appreciation extends to the many patients, clinicians, and researchers who continue to inspire us with their commitment to advancing healthcare using technology. We thank the broader AI and pharmaceutical communities for their ongoing dedication to improving patient outcomes and pushing the boundaries of what is possible in medicine. Also, I especially acknowledge Ravi Teja Kothuru for his contributions to this work.

Competing Interests The authors have no competing interests to declare that are relevant to the content of this manuscript.

Contents

List of Figures

List of Tables

1 Introduction to Artificial Intelligence in Pharmaceutical Sciences

Artificial intelligence is rapidly emerging as a defining force in the pharmaceutical sciences, promising to revolutionize every aspect from basic research to clinical application. This technological transformation is rooted in the convergence of vast biomedical datasets, powerful computational resources, and sophisticated algorithms capable of learning, reasoning, and autonomous decision-making. As the pharmaceutical industry faces mounting pressure to innovate and accelerate drug development, AI offers a unique toolkit to overcome longstanding challenges, enabling researchers to discover new therapeutics, optimize clinical trials, and personalize patient care with unprecedented speed and precision. In this chapter, we embark on an exploration of AI's origins, principles, and its remarkable journey into the heart of pharmaceutical science.

1.1 Overview of AI and Machine Learning

Artificial intelligence (AI) and machine learning (ML) technologies have transformed several scientific fields and will transform across scientific disciplines, especially drug discovery. AI and ML permit the identification of data-driven learning, cognitive learning processes, and task-learning automation. The objective of this section is to provide a broad overview of AI and ML, from its conceptual inspirations to the foundational and recent developments that inform their use in drug discovery.

K. Shaikh et al., *Artificial Intelligence in Drug Discovery and Development*,
Synthesis Lectures on Engineering, Science, and Technology,
https://doi.org/10.1007/978-3-032-10277-5_1

1.1.1 Definition of Artificial Intelligence

Artificial intelligence (AI) can be explained as the simulation of human intelligence by machines programmed to think and learn (n.d.) [1]. AI involves many different subfields such as natural language processing (NLP), computer vision, expert systems, and robotics, but specifically ML and DL. During drug discovery AI is important in predicting molecular properties, virtual screening, de novo drug design, and target identification (G.M.C. Hall et al., n.d.) [2].

The term "AI" was first used at the Dartmouth Conference in 1956 and has since made historical shifts from various phases of optimism, disenchantment, and resurgence largely due to increases in computational power and real-world data availability [3]. Each wave of AI advancement had many cycles or "AI winters" characterized by a lack of real-world success in the first few decades due to weak data and the limitations of hardware. However, the last decade, specifically since 2010, has propelled the field of AI to unprecedented momentum in drug-related applications due to deep learning breakthroughs and because of an exponential increase in biological and chemical datasets.

AI is now used in drug discovery to help with molecular docking simulations, high-throughput screening (HTS) optimization, and compound similarity searching. Expert systems provide chemists with decision support while executing lead optimization. AI-based robotic systems are also utilized to automate synthesis, test compounds, and annotate data. This means that we now have sophisticated types of AI technologies that accelerate the progression of potential drug compounds to this valuable hit-to-lead stage [2].

1.1.2 Understanding of Machine Learning

Machine learning (ML), a subdomain of AI, is defined as the ability of systems to learn from experience and adapt automatically, without being explicitly programmed. ML algorithms can learn the structure of the data through training from historical data and to build predictive models and make decisions on new input data [4]. As shown in Fig. 1.1, the commonly used definitions of the different types of ML are as follows:

- **Supervised Learning:** Algorithms are trained on labeled data (e.g., drug classification or toxicity prediction). The goal of the algorithms is to learn a mapping from some input features to a target label. Many branches of supervised learning use an objective function, such as mean squared error or cross-entropy loss to optimize the model.
- **Unsupervised Learning:** This is popular for working with unlabeled data to find underlying distributions in data (e.g., clustering of molecules). Some of the most well-known unsupervised learning tools are K-means clustering, PCA, and autoencoders that enable data visualization, data compression, and identification of anomalies.

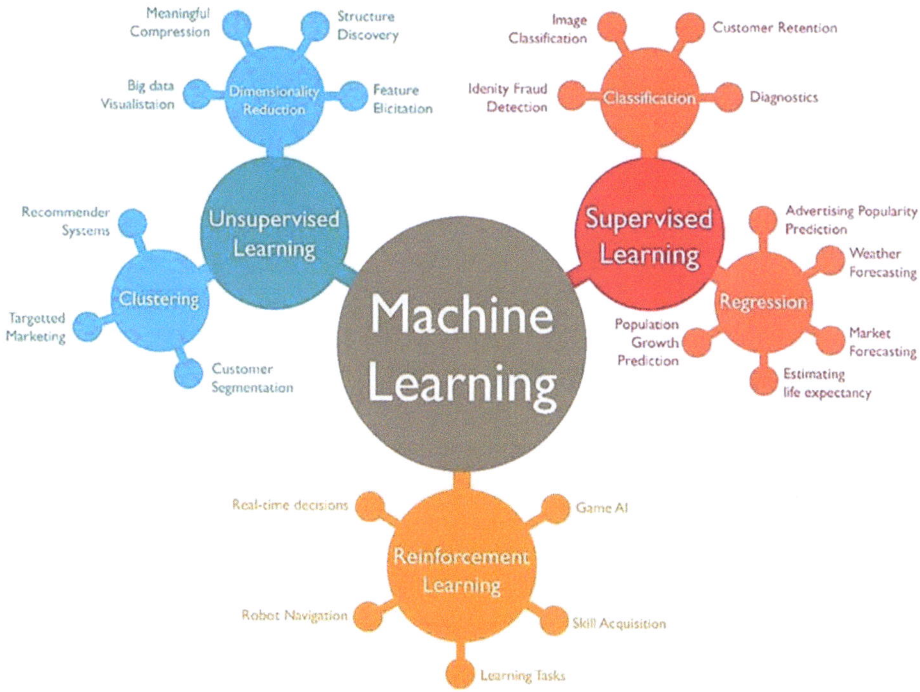

Fig. 1.1 Different types of machine learning

- **Reinforcement Learning:** Reinforcement learning trains algorithms on an optimal action through trial and error (e.g., generating molecules with desired pharmacological profiles). These methods are best suited for stochastic decision-making problems described by Markov decision processes. Reinforcement learning is gaining interest in contexts, e.g., adaptive trial designs or robotics automation.

In the pharmaceutical space, supervised ML predicts bioactivity of molecules, unsupervised ML clusters compounds with similar properties, and reinforcement learning can now be used in de novo drug generation. Ensemble methods also provide robust predictions in the face of uncertainty along with probabilistic learning models in a handful of circumstances [4, 5]. Further, there exists a strong relationship with ML, statistical inference, and optimization. Gradient descent and variations thereof (e.g., stochastic gradient descent) are work-horse algorithms used to train many modern ML models. Loss functions, regularization, and hyperparameter optimization (grid search or Bayesian optimization) often weigh heavily on the ability of a model to generalize.

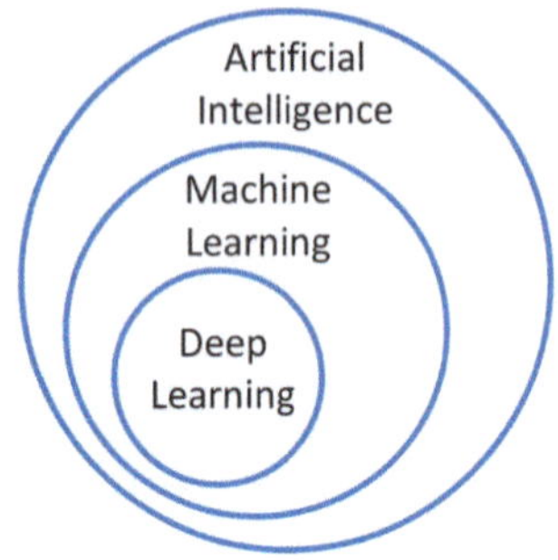

Fig. 1.2 Conceptual hierarchy of AI, ML, and DL

1.1.3 Deep Learning and Its Role

Deep learning, which is a subset of machine learning as shown in Fig. 1.2, employs deep neural networks to identify higher level features from the raw data [6]. Deep learning has been successful in working with complex unstructured data types such as image, text, and biological sequence data [7]. Deep learning has disrupted protein structure prediction in the form of AlphaFold [8], and rapidly identifying kinase inhibitors [9] makes it stand out from other machine learning techniques.

1.1.4 Various AI Algorithms Used in Pharmaceutical Sciences

The pharmaceutical sciences apply many of the various AI algorithms well-known as shown in Table 1.1 [10–12].

1.1.5 The Fuel for Model Learning Training (Data)

AI systems are always reliant on data. In the pharmaceutical industry or drug discovery, that data includes molecular structure, pharmacokinetics, genomic sequencing, patient demographics, drug structures, clinical trials, adverse events, and real-world evidence (see Fig. 1.3). Each type of data can introduce unique challenges and opportunities in the application of AI; on the one hand, high-throughput screening (HTS) datasets are massive but might contain inconsistencies; electronic health records (EHRs) contain extensive patient context but can be noisy and unstructured [4].

The preprocessing of this diversity of data is important. Consistent processes such as normalization, tokenization (in the case of textual data), and encoding (e.g., SMILES strings for molecular data) are all necessary to prepare it to ingest into machine learning (ML) pipelines. Equally important are dimensionality reduction processes, like principal component analysis (PCA) and t-distributed stochastic neighbor embedding (t-SNE) to combat the curse of dimensionality and improve interpretability of models.

Table 1.1 Various AI algorithms used in pharmaceutical science

Algorithm	Description	Pharmaceutical use cases
Decision trees	Classification is based on rules	ADMET prediction
Random forest	This is based on ensemble learning methods	Drug response modeling
Support vector machines	Classification happens with hyperplans having maximum margins	Compound activity prediction
Neural networks (NNs)	Inspired by brain neurons and works with multilayered perceptrons	Protein-ligand interaction modeling
Convolutional neural networks (CNNs)	Neural networks specializes for spatial data	Image-based screening and tissue recognition
Recurrent neural networks (RNNs)	Neural networks specializes for temporal data processing	Time-series analysis of clinical trials

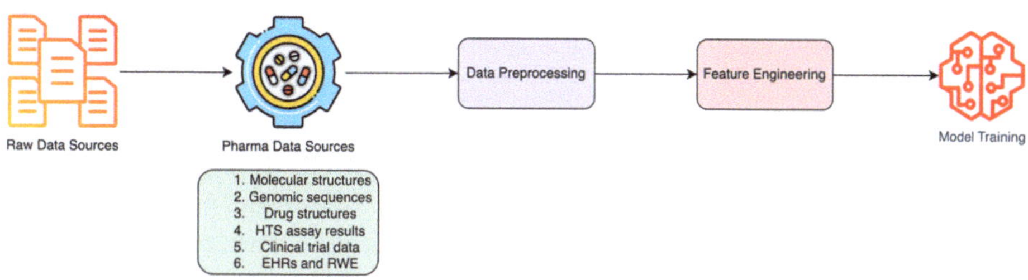

Fig. 1.3 Data fuel for model learning in drug discovery

Models also need to implement methods to deal with missing and imbalanced data, both of which are common sets of issues in pharmaceutical datasets. Some methods like data imputation, SMOTE (as syntactic multimodal oversampling), and data augmentation help with the robustness to data while also reducing bias [13].

1.1.6 Feature Engineering Vs. Representation Learning

Feature engineering relies on human selection, transformation, and generation of variables (i.e., features) to better model performance. It is iterative, reliant on domain expertise, and time-consuming, but it was the state of the art before DL [4]. In pharmaceutical sciences, companies could select and generate descriptors such as molecular weight, lipophilicity logP ratios, topological polar surface area, and so on.

On the other hand, representation learning, mainly through DL models, is automated. For example, word embeddings (e.g., Word2Vec in the biomedical literature), graph neural networks (GNNs for molecular graphs), and convolutional layers (for biomedical images) can learn patterns and abstractions from raw forms of data [6]. The process of representation learning provides the opportunity for a researcher to circumvent the process of manual feature crafting and allow for exploration of rich unstructured high dimensional data.

Representation learning is one of the many building blocks for addressing complex problems, such as AlphaFold, which revolutionized protein structure determination by converting a sequence of amino acids to a 3D structural representation using a DL architecture [8]. Other generative models, such as variational autoencoders (VAEs) and generative adversarial networks (GANs), have opened a pathway for de novo molecular design and the richness of capturing complex interactions between features that are ignored by contemporary models. The decision to use feature engineering or representation learning often depends on the size of the data, nature of the task, and computational resources available. In practice, hybrid approaches with a mix of domain-informed features and learned embeddings are best practice in many pharmaceutical AI pipelines.

1.1.7 Summary of Conceptual Landscape

If you see Table 1.2, examining the transition AI creates for pharmaceutical sciences can help us evaluate the differences between traditional computational approaches and AI-based systems in a few important areas. A traditional approach has been built on deterministic, rule-based logic, which must be defined by human rules and features. The traditional approach rarely could successfully scale or adapt to new information or environments. In contrast, AI- and ML-based approaches leverage statistical learning, probabilistic inference, and enormous parallelism—such that an AI system will build and adapt as new data are available while improving feedback mechanisms in the original onboard data. For instance, the traditional QSAR models must undergo feature selection in a rigorous manner, whereas DL can take molecular graphs (which are not only raw and based on multiple types of information) and assess structure-activity relationships without direct instruction [5, 6].

Table 1.2 Transition AI creates for pharmaceutical sciences

Dimension	Traditional approach	ML approach
Knowledge derivation	Expert rules	Data-driven learning
Feature extraction	Manual	Automated (representation learning)
Prediction capability	Limited	High accuracy with large-scale data
Scalability	Low	High
Adaptability	Static	Dynamic and self-improving
Generalization	Task-specific	Transferable across domains
Model complexity	Low	High (deep architectures)

1.1.8 Key Terminology

For effective use of AI literature in the field of pharmaceutical sciences, clarity regarding terminology is critical. Many terms referenced in AI literature have overlapping definitions and contexts of implementation.

- **Artificial Intelligence (AI):** Refers to systems which mimic the cognitive abilities of humans such as learning, reasoning, and self-correction [1].
- **Machine Learning (ML):** A subdomain of AI which deals with algorithms utilizing data to improve their model performance over iterations of data collection [6].
- **Deep Learning (DL):** A subdomain of ML which uses multilayer neural networks designed to learn abstract representations [6].
- **Neural Networks (NN):** Composed of individual nodes (or neurons) located in multiple layers with connection weights, to allow the processing of an input matrix [6].
- **Reinforcement Learning (RL):** A framework in which agents learn to act in a way that maximizes cumulative reward for whatever optimization objective that means, often useful for sequential decision-making [4].
- **Supervised Learning:** Works with labeled dataset, focuses on supporting classifying objects, regression, etc. [10].
- **Unsupervised Learning:** Works with unlabeled datasets to find patterns or groupings inherent to the data [10].

1.2 Historical Context of AI in Healthcare

The employment of artificial intelligence (AI) in the healthcare sector is not a novel idea; it has developed over years of collaborative developments, advances in computational systems, and the need for improved clinical outcomes. The growth of artificial intelligence in healthcare has always had a mix of early theoretical considerations, experiences, and a desire to improve clinical outcomes while being efficient in organizational performance. This part of the book will outline the story of AI in healthcare by identifying moments in history, changes in paradigm, and emergent changes.

1.2.1 The Genesis (1950s–1970s)

As shown in Table 1.3, the conceptual foundation of AI dates to the mid-twentieth century. Alan Turing introduced the idea of machine intelligence and the well-known Turing test in 1950 and posited whether machines can think like people [14, 15]. The term "artificial intelligence" was coined in 1956 at the Dartmouth Summer Research Project on Artificial Intelligence, laying the educational and research groundwork for the field [14–16].

Table 1.3 Early AI milestones in healthcare

Year	AI milestone
1950	Turing test
1956	Dartmouth conference
1960s	Early pattern recognition in medicine
1971	INTERNIST-1
1976	MYCIN

Between 1960 and 1970, we saw initial exploratory applications of AI in health. To begin, we saw the emergence of INTERNIST-1 in 1971, which began the era of computerized clinical decision support, using search algorithms to help with differential diagnosis [16]. Shortly after, MYCIN emerged, which was a rule-based expert system, and recommended antibiotic treatments for bacterial infections. MYCIN led the way for AI use in medical reasoning and therapy selection [14, 16, 17].

Some of these early systems were limited by the computational capability and access to data in the time window. However, they manifested the paradigm for future AI-based diagnostic and decision support tools [18].

1.2.2 Further Expansion and Experimentation

The infusion of expert systems and AI into clinical workflows characterized the 1980s and 1990s. As an example, DXplain (University of Massachusetts, 1986) built on the capabilities of INTERNIST-1, which allowed clinicians to enter symptoms, and potentially receive additional diagnoses. These systems were also beginning to function as initial information banks for current medical knowledge. AI's function in clinical medicine continued to expand beyond diagnosis into the clinical areas of medical imaging, surgical assistance, and managing electronic health record (EHR) data [17]. For example, AI-enabled algorithms created faster data collection and processing, enhanced the accuracy of surgical functions, and allowed EHRs to be implemented to a greater extent [17]. In 1989, Cedars-Sinai first utilized CorSage as an AI intervention to help identify heart patients who are at risk of suffering recurrent coronary events—this would be the beginning of risk stratification through AI [15]. Figure 1.4 shows the evolution of AI in healthcare systems.

Despite the possibilities for AI development and deployment, there was still an inherent slow uptake of AI due to limiting factors such as the ability to access computational power or resources, the complexities of medical data, and the validation of an AI algorithm in clinical practice [18].

1.2.3 The 2000s Digital Revolution

If you see Table 1.4, the early twenty-first century was a pivotal moment in the history of AI in healthcare. The dance of events began with the expansion of electronic health

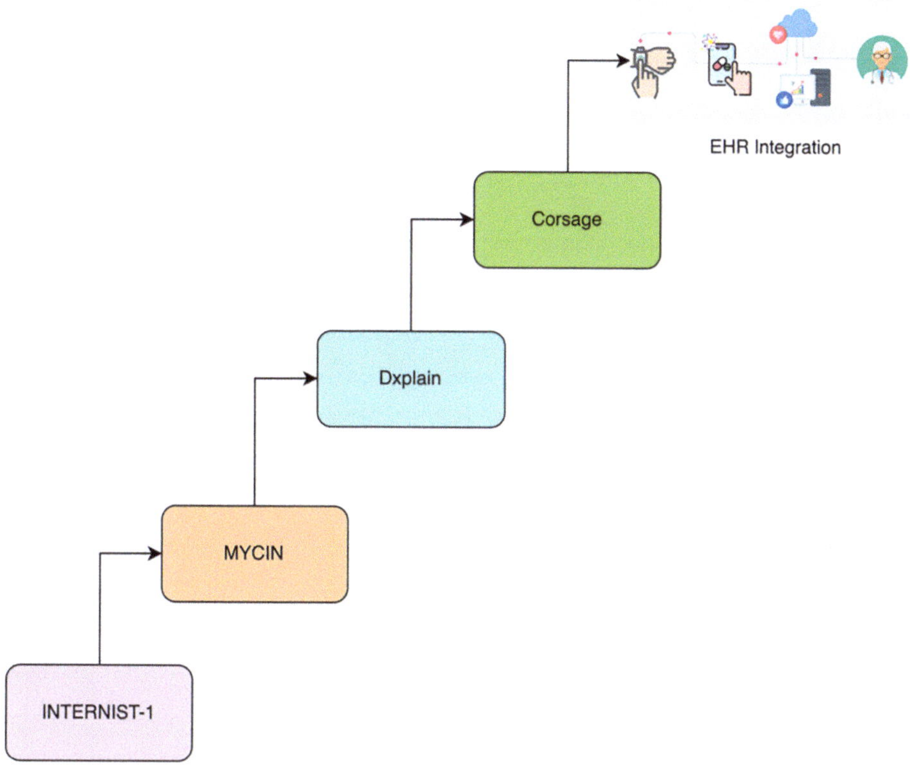

Fig. 1.4 Evolution of AI systems in healthcare (1970–1990s) [15–17]

Table 1.4 Key Developments in healthcare AI during the 2000s

Year	AI milestone
2000s	EHR adoption and ML integration
2003	Genome human project completion
2007	IBM Watson (DeepQA)

records (EHR), advances in hardware processing, vast amounts of medical records, and the development of machine learning (ML) algorithms [14, 15, 19]. This marked the beginning of the journey of ML, which is an expansion of AI that focuses on data-driven recognition of patterns. AI and ML systems utilized early prototypes to analyze EHR data, medical imaging, and genomics data before maturing analytic capabilities have emerged [14, 18].

The adoption of EHR in clinical facilities produced a broad swath of structured and unstructured data, which, in aggregate, was a veritable replication for exploitation of ML technologies [15, 19]. AI systems began to be operationalized to analyze EHRs, images, and genome data, enabling clinical care to better informed/diagnosed patients, use risk stratification protocols, and better patient management overall [14, 18, 20].

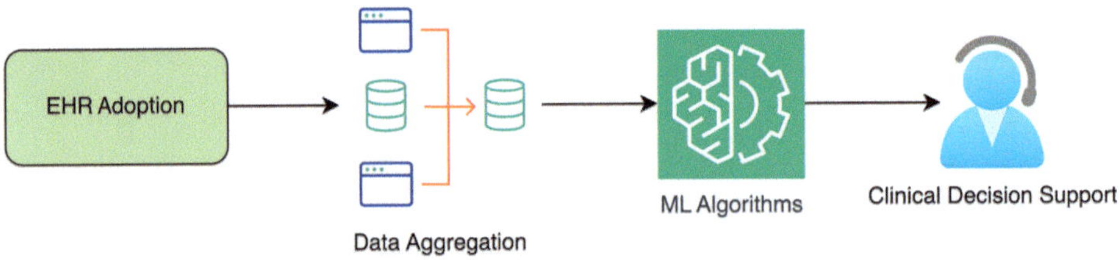

Fig. 1.5 AI Integration workflow in healthcare

The emergence of big data analytics allowed heterogeneous datasets to processed/analyzed/interpreted by AI systems at substantial scale, for instance (as shown in Fig. 1.5), the ability for AI algorithms to automatically extract clinical information from EHR datasets, identify patterns of populations, or forecast regional disease outbreaks [14, 18].

These developments set the groundwork for the next era of AI in healthcare, the deep learning revolution. However, issues remained. Data quality, interoperability, and privacy issues often limited the utility of early AI systems [17, 19] and the interpretability of ML models, particularly those utilizing complex statistical methods, remained an impediment to clinical trust and adoption [21, 22].

1.2.4 The Deep Learning Era: 2010s

The 2010s marked the beginning of the period of deep learning, which is a specialized feature of ML based on multilayer neural networks that model the complex, nonlinear relationships found in data [18, 21, 23]. A series of advances in deep learning systems and methodologies lead to life-changing breakthroughs in the domain of healthcare AI.

- **Medical Imaging**. The performance of deep learning algorithms exceeded that of traditional statistical methods and, in many cases, simply matched or exceeded that of human experts. Deep learning algorithms, with convolutional neural networks (CNNs) at the forefront, were reported to have achieved human-level performance (in addition to labeled datasets of hundreds of thousands of images) for examples of detecting diabetic retinopathies in retinal images [23], identifying lung cancer in CT scans [20], and classifying skin lesions [24]. The power of deep learning to extract small, subtle diagnostic features from high-dimensional data has contributed to a revolution in diagnostic radiology and pathology [21, 25].
- **Natural Language Processing**. Similar advances in natural language processing (NLP) also occurred that allowed AI systems to extract actionable insights from unstructured clinical notes, scholarly research articles, and biomedical literature [17, 20, 21] AI-enabled NLP tools could automate the summarization of patient history, alert users of potential adverse interactions, and promote new knowledge discovery from the vastness of medical text [18, 21].

- **Predictive Analytics and Personalized Medicine**. The incorporation of deep learning into the mix of clinical and genomic data created predictive analytics. AI tools could now provide predictions of disease progression, identify high-risk patients, and suggest personalized treatment protocols [14, 19, 21] for chronic diseases. One clinical usage of deep learning included predicting the onset of sepsis, heart failure, and long-term critical illness based on electronic health record (EHR) data and models trained on imaging data from the EHRs [18, 21, 23].

The expansion of readily available open-source deep learning frameworks and large annotated datasets has also opened access to great AI tools [23, 26]. The collaboration of academia backed by industry and needing intervention/innovation has provided a lactation for predictive analytics and AI to thrive to the benefit of human health and recovery [14, 17, 18]. Nonetheless, the rapid uptake of deep learning elaborated new potential challenges. Model interpretability, data privacy, and algorithm bias have become high profile issues [21, 22, 25]. A consideration directed toward building AI systems that improved interpretability, fairness, and generalizability across diverse populations became a research and regulatory focus [18, 19, 21]. The timeline of AI milestones in healthcare is shown in Fig. 1.6.

1.2.5 AI in the Modern Clinic (2020s)

Over the last decade, AI has become part of the delivery of healthcare, including applications of AI in diagnostics, treatment planning, operational effectiveness, and patient engagement [21, 27, 28]. AI-powered tools now assist clinicians with medical imaging interpretation, predicting outcome of patients, and automating administrative functions [20].

- **Dramatic Expansion of Application**. The COVID-19 pandemic drastically increased the implementation of AI in healthcare, as the need for rapid diagnostics, resource allocation, and remote monitoring emerged [15, 18, 29]. AI models were used for the projections of outbreak trajectory, optimized testing strategies, and aided the development of vaccines [16, 21, 28].

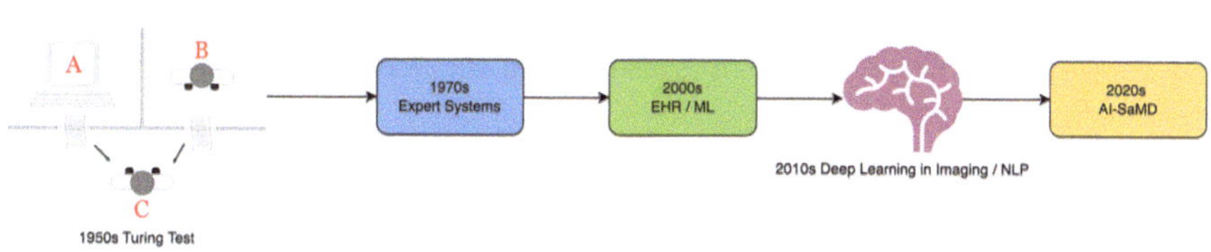

Fig. 1.6 Timeline of AI milestones in healthcare (1950s–2020s) [14, 15, 19, 21, 23]

Table 1.5 Examples of AI integration in modern healthcare

Domain	Example application
Diagnostics	Automated imaging analysis
Treatment planning	Precision oncology
Operations	Resource allocation
Patient engagement	Virtual health assistants

- **AI in Clinical Practice**. AI is being integrated into multiple facets of everyday clinical practice. In radiology, AI-based diagnostic tools detect abnormalities in X-rays and MRIs; pathology applications analyze biopsy slides; and cardiology models interpret electrocardiograms [18, 20, 21, 23]. In oncology, AI models facilitate precision medicine by utilizing genomic, imaging, and clinical data to recommend treatment selection [19, 25, 26].

AI is also supporting operational elements of healthcare, including workflow optimization in hospitals and clinics, as well as improved scheduling and resource allocation [18, 24, 29]. Further, virtual assistants and chatbots enhance patient engagement through education, appointment reminders, and symptom triage [17, 18]. While many advances have been made in the adoption of AI in healthcare, many challenges remain. Notably, continuing to ensure generalizability of AI models, data privacy concerns, and the ethical considerations continue to be high priority topics for researchers, clinicians, and detection of healthcare inequities [5, 23, 24, 28].

As shown in Table 1.5, the historical context surrounding AI in healthcare illustrates a path from early rule-based expert systems, through the current period of deep learning and integrated clinical decision support, and has included capabilities, challenges, and opportunities in each decade so far, eventually leading to widespread adoption of AI in the existing healthcare system. Although AI continues to grow and has the potential to improve patient outcomes, improve operational efficiency, and drive medical innovation, its benefits can only be realized if ethical, regulatory, and technical challenges are approached thoughtfully [14, 17, 25, 27].

1.3 Importance of AI in Drug Discovery and Development

Artificial intelligence (AI) has the potential to redesign the pharmaceutical sciences, especially in drug discovery and development aspects. AI can analyze vast datasets, simulate molecular interactions, predict therapeutic efficacy, and provide a new approach to an entire pharmaceutical pipeline. AI is transforming the way new drugs are discovered, developed, and deployed [30–32].

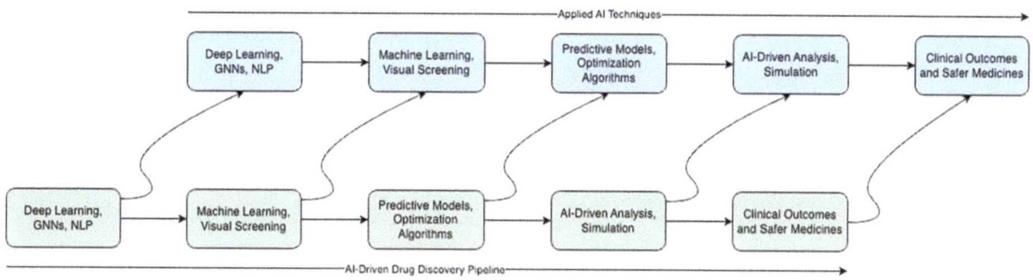

Fig. 1.7 AI Drug discovery pipeline [32]

1.3.1 Accelerating Drug Discovery

Drug discovery processes often take many years or even a decade; costs are extraordinary. As shown in Fig. 1.7, AI changes the way that pharmaceutical scientists undertake the early parts of drug discovery—including target identification, lead compound selection, and structure-based drug design. Trained algorithms using machine learning applications can identify possible drug candidates in a fraction of the time by identifying patterns in large datasets of chemical structures and biological outcomes [32–34].

For example, artificial intelligence (AI) methods such as generative adversarial networks (GANs) and variational autoencoders allow scientists to create novel molecular structures that have desirable biological properties [35]. The high content and high-throughput screening data can be analyzed and novel insights gained from deep learning models like convolutional neural networks (CNNs) and recurrent neural networks (RNNs) [36, 37].

Deep learning models have shown enormous value in drug repurposing that is, using deep learning to map the relationships between drugs and disease to identify new purposes for existing drugs using transcriptome and proteome data [38, 39]. For example, AI-assisted discovery of DDR1 kinase inhibitors using deep learning approaches resulted in previously unidentified inhibitors with substantial potency [39].

1.3.2 Enhancing Efficiency in Drug Development

As shown in Fig. 1.8, artificial intelligence (AI) has substantial impact in the optimization of the development phase of drug discovery where AI can be used in various applications [33] (see Fig. 1.9) such as optimizing clinical trials designs, enhanced patient recruitment, and evaluating clinical outcomes in a real-time basis [33, 38]. Other areas of development that can be achieved with machine learning models during development is to predict drug efficacy and toxicity which can help decrease the probability of late-stage failure [31, 32].

Natural language processing (NLP) techniques have enabled the mining of scientific literature along with electronic health records (EHRs) to generate inferred insights regarding adverse drug reactions, contraindications, and real-world outcomes [40, 41]. The

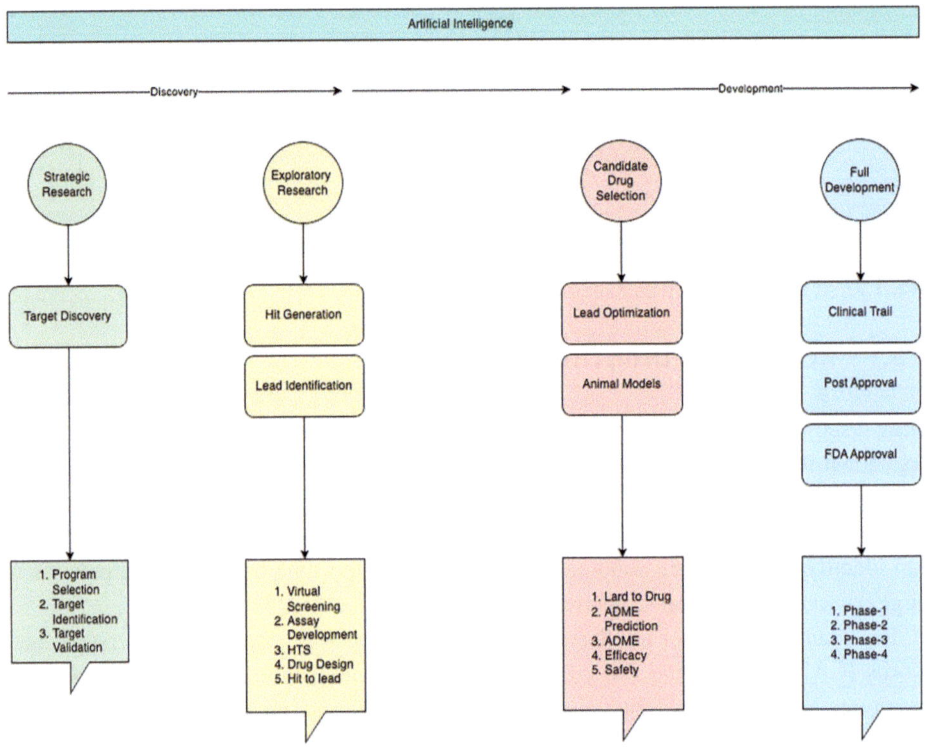

Fig. 1.8 AI extends drug discovery to development phases [31]

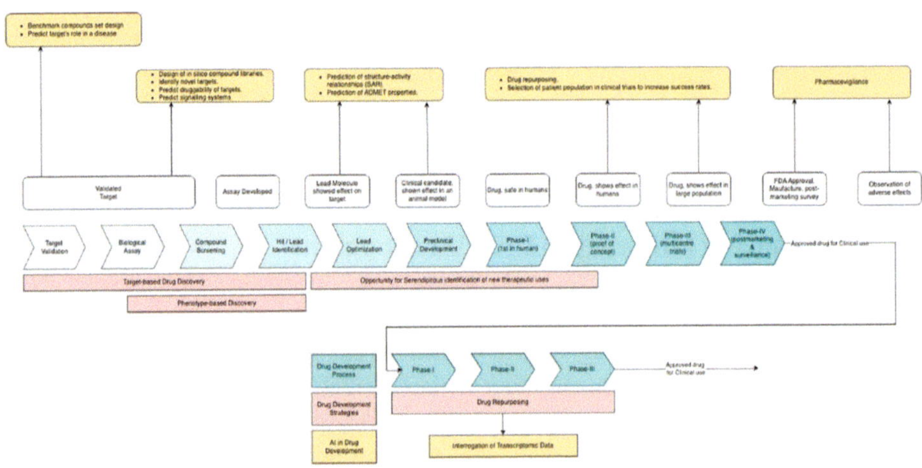

Fig. 1.9 Applications of AI across drug development pipeline [33]

application of predictive modeling techniques can help lead in identifying optimal dosing regimens and the evaluation of pharmacokinetics/pharmacodynamics (PK/PD) parameters, therefore enabling faster transitions between bench and bedside [42].

1.3.3 Drug Design and Molecular Development

One of the potential cornerstones of AI in pharmaceutical R&D is its ability to create drug-like small molecules from scratch. In generative models, like druGAN (a GAN-based architecture), the model is trained to generate molecules with desired biological properties to fit predefined biological targets [35]. AI models also simulate molecular docking (as shown in Fig. 1.10) and optimize lead compounds with scoring functions to limit trial-and-error experiments in lab [32, 37]. There are existing tools (i.e., DeepChem, GravNet, and MolGAN) that can leverage a generative model to create and score large libraries of drug-like molecules for drug-likeness, binding affinity, and toxicity profile [43]. Additionally, generative models use transfer learning and reinforcement learning to further fine-tune the generative model for domain-specific optimization [37, 44].

1.3.4 Predictive Toxicology and ADMET Modeling

As shown in Fig. 1.11, toxicity and suboptimal pharmacokinetic profiles constitute one of the top reasons behind drug development failures and late-state trial terminations are extremely costly. AI provides a powerful mechanism for toxicology predictions and modeling ADMET (absorption, distribution, metabolism, excretion, and toxicity) using in silico means [10, 33, 42]. AI models thrive on historical toxicology data and predictive toxicity models using ensemble methods, such as random forests and gradient boosting machines, and perform well at predicting adverse effects, bioaccumulation, and toxicity to specific organs [40, 43].

In addition to ensemble methods, various advanced deep learning architectures [33] can utilize chemical structure descriptor and fingerprints to model nonlinear relationships in

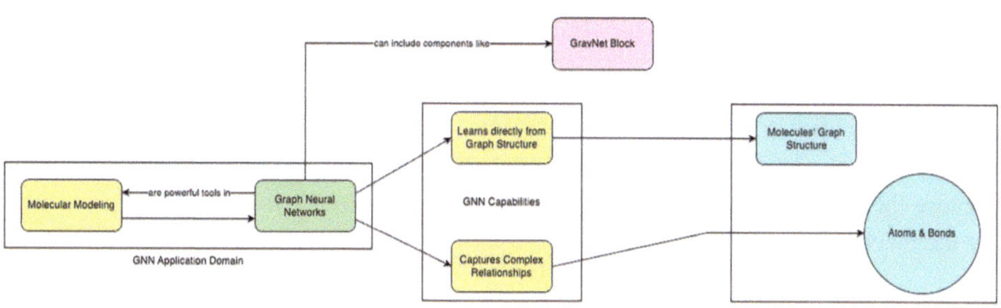

Fig. 1.10 Molecular modeling using GravNet [32]

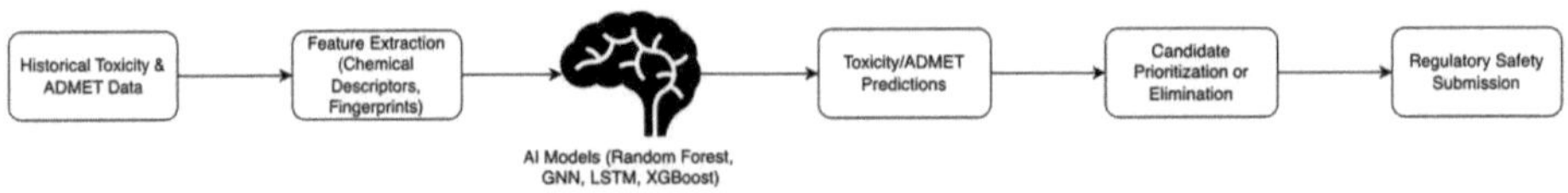

Fig. 1.11 AI-enabled predictive toxicology pipeline

the complex datasets typically seen in toxicity data. For example, long short-term memory (LSTM) and graph neural networks (GNNs) have been successfully utilized to identify compounds that inhibit hERG channel function, whereby hERG channel function is a critical cardiac safety element of the drug development process [32]. Moreover, having ADMET profiles aided by AI models reduces dependence on animal studies, as well as removing unviable drug candidates in the early phases of drug development, meaning improved downstream productivity as well [33]. The FDA and EMA have also shown increasing interest in allowing the use of validated AI models as part of a regulatory submission for safety information [41].

1.3.5 AI and Robotics Integration in Drug Discovery

The incorporation of AI into robotics is producing advances in automation and throughput never seen in the field of drug discovery. Self-driving laboratories encompassing robotic arms, automated liquid handlers, and AI-driven decision systems are transforming how we think about experimentation [34, 45].

These systems work together to autonomously design, perform, and analyze high-throughput experimentations. For example, an AI model can analyze the results of assays in real time and determine the next experimental conditions using reinforcement learning algorithms [33]. The closed loop allows for real-time updates and serves to test and reassess new hypotheses without the need for human intervention, enabling trial and error in lead optimization cycles to happen at unprecedented speeds. Cobots are being utilized for tasks such as, but not limited to, compound synthesis, parallel screening, and live cell imaging [34].

Meanwhile, AI-powered robotic platform screening has provided viable solutions to global crises in healthcare over the last few years, where parts or mechanisms, like the need to quickly screen hundreds to thousands of antiviral compounds during the progression of the COVID-19 pandemic, have allowed for scalable solutions during periods of urgency. The ability to quickly perform multiple iterations in drug screening makes robotic platforms ideal platforms for the study and treatment of rare diseases and conditions because there are often few samples available and precision plays a vital role in elucidating the mechanisms of action. See Fig. 1.12 for better understanding.

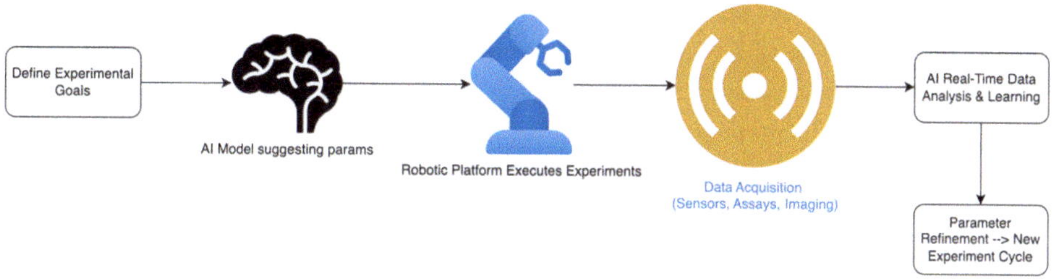

Fig. 1.12 AI-robotics workflow in automated drug screening

1.3.6 Clinical Trial Optimization

Clinical trials are one of the most cost-intensive and time-intensive aspects of drug development. AI can optimize the clinical trial process regarding design, subject selection, and monitoring in real time. Stratification of patients with AI tools also enables identification of participants who are genetically or phenotypically appropriate for the trial. This selection of genetically or phenotypically appropriate participants improves the likelihood of detection of a treatment response and reduces unpredictability across participating subjects [31, 33, 41].

AI has tremendous potential to assess multimodal datasets, including electronic health records (EHRs), genomics, proteomics, and patient-reported outcomes, and to match patients to the trial that best fits their profile [38]. Additionally, predictive models predict key trial metrics regarding speed of enrollment, rate of dropout, and likelihood of meeting a primary endpoint to make amendments to trial protocols proactively, if necessary [33].

AI has also enhanced natural language processing tools to extract and summarize actionable trial information from unstructured data sources, including clinical notes, pathology reports, and literature databases [40]. Also, wearable biosensors with AI allow investigators to continuously monitor patients and provide real-time feedback [42]. After experiencing the pandemic, virtual trials (or hybrid trials) utilizing AI for decentralized data capture has gained traction and show potential to enhance patient engagement while reducing operational costs [41, 44].

1.3.7 Challenges and Ethical Considerations

The application of AI in drug development is enormous, but the application of AI to drug development is not without challenges. One of the biggest challenges is the interpretability of AI models. Many deep learning models survive on their performance but suffer from limitations. Even when deep learning models predict accurately, they often function in black boxes that don't easily convey what caused the report [40, 46]. While regulations agencies want to review the number of models submitted and reports provided (essentially confirming accuracy), they also want a clear rationale used to make the safety-related decision.

Further concerns exist regarding data quality and representativeness, the numbers that provide the license for AI models or predictions. AI models are only as good as the data prepared to train. Datasets are frequently biased, whether they are demographic, ethnic, or biological originating from and are falsely representational, or introduce unintended predictions and impacts. Additionally, the absence of data and/or training from larger datasets or substandard representation will limit the ability of an AI model to generalize across different populations or areas of disease.

There is a range of ethical implications, from the potential misuse of AI-generated molecules for premeditated harm to the questionable use of patient data and privacy. It is vital to ensure safe and anonymous use of this data to protect trust and compliance with laws and regulations [40]. To answer these concerns, the field is shifting to explainable AI (XAI) models, which provide insight into the reasoning and justification for predictions. The FDA and EMA are establishing pathways for the validation and certification of AI tools that are intended for use in drug development [32, 41]. It will take collaboration across the fields of computer science, clinical medicine, ethics, and regulatory affairs to create an empirically reliable, safe, and ethical AI ecosphere.

1.3.8 The Future Outlook of AI in Drug Discovery and Development

In the future, the added strength from AI interacting with quantum computing, blockchain, and multi-omic platforms will continue to enhance the capabilities of drug discovery [30, 31]. Explainable AI (XAI) models are becoming popular as models that you can make predictions transparently and interpretable. In addition, federated learning is becoming a popular alternative for handling data privacy, allowing model building among institutions without disclosing personal data [40, 44]. There is an ever-increasing collaboration in the pharmaceutical ecosystem, and together, academia, industry, and regulators will continue to use AI ethically and responsibly [32, 33].

1.4 Current Applications of Artificial Intelligence in Pharmaceutical Sciences

The traditional drug discovery and development pipeline is long (≈10–15 years) and costly (≈USD 1–2 billion per new drug) with a very low clinical success rate (fewer than 1 in 10 candidates entering Phase I eventually approved) [47]. AI and ML methods are being applied at every stage of this pipeline—from target identification and hit finding through lead optimization and ADMET profiling to trial simulation and design—with the goal of increasing speed and success rates. Unlike sequential workflows, AI can integrate diverse data (genomic, proteomic, chemical, clinical) in parallel, potentially compressing years of preclinical work into months. In target identification, for example, AI-based tools use text mining of the literature, multi-omics analyses, network pharmacology, and chemical similarity to uncover disease-relevant targets that may be missed by classical methods. Such approaches include natural language processing (NLP) on biomedical texts, graph neural networks on protein-protein or gene networks, and ML on transcriptomic/proteomic profiles. In one survey, transformer-based "Mol-BERT" models pre-trained on millions of molecules have been used to capture latent chemical rules for target prediction, while graph neural nets have achieved very high accuracy (e.g., AUC $\approx$ 0.96) in drug-target interaction tasks [47, 48]. More generally, AI models can analyze vast public databases of genomics and pathway data to flag novel targets and biomarkers for disease.

AI-driven computational chemistry and de novo design methods are rapidly transforming lead discovery and optimization. Deep learning and generative models can propose novel small molecules with desired properties, greatly expanding the explorable chemical space. Leading AI biotech companies have demonstrated concrete successes. For example, **Insilico Medicine** identified a new target and brought a candidate for idiopathic pulmonary fibrosis into preclinical trials within 18 months at a cost of only ~$150,000 (versus ~4–6 years traditionally). **Exscientia**, in partnership with Sumitomo Pharma, used AI-driven design to create DSP-1181 (for OCD) in under 12 months—the first AI-designed molecule to enter human trials. **Recursion Pharmaceuticals** combines automated high-content cell imaging with deep learning to detect phenotypic drug effects, enabling rapid repurposing and discovery of novel therapeutics. **Schrödinger's** platform integrates physics-based molecular simulation with AI to predict protein-ligand interactions, significantly improving virtual screening hit rates [47]. Such examples illustrate that AI can substantially shorten discovery timelines and reduce experimental costs. Across many therapeutic areas, reported studies find that classical ML methods predominate ($\approx$41%), with physics simulations ($\approx$21%) and deep learning ($\approx$10%) also widely used [47]. Although oncology remains a major focus ($\approx$73% of studies), AI methods are increasingly applied to diverse diseases. By coupling AI predictions with high-throughput automated synthesis and screening, the industry aims to move from serendipitous discovery to rational, AI-guided design.

1.4.1 AI in Clinical Trials

AI is also impacting clinical development by optimizing trial design, improving recruitment and monitoring, and predicting outcomes. A recent review found hundreds of AI/ML studies applied to clinical trial **risk assessment** (safety, efficacy, and operational risks) [48]. AI algorithms (including traditional ML, deep learning, and causal methods) can analyze large volumes of data—from electronic health records and genomic profiles to historical trial databases—to flag safety signals or side effect risks more efficiently than manual methods. For instance, models trained on preclinical and early clinical data can predict the likelihood of toxicity or treatment failure, potentially allowing early trial termination of unsafe or ineffective drug candidates. In one survey of recent work, some AI models achieved AUROC ≈0.96 in retrospective trial outcome prediction, though issues of bias and data quality remain. Beyond risk assessment, AI is being deployed to improve operational aspects of trials. Machine learning can identify eligible patients from health records and social media, optimizing recruitment to match patients with appropriate trials. Generative and NLP models may help design better protocols or consent forms. In silico trial simulators (virtual twins) use patient data and mechanistic models to forecast outcomes under different trial designs. Overall, AI-driven tools promise to streamline trial planning, patient stratification, and real-time monitoring—increasing trial efficiency and reducing costs [48].

1.4.2 AI in Personalized Medicine

Personalized (precision) medicine—tailoring therapies to an individual's genetic, molecular, and clinical profile—is a major application area for AI. Modern patient datasets (genomes, transcriptomes, metabolomes) are high-dimensional and complex; AI/ML methods excel at finding predictive patterns in such data. Recently, **generative AI** (GANs, VAEs, etc.) has emerged as a promising approach. A systematic review of generative AI in personalized medicine (549 screened studies) identified 27 relevant examples: most used GANs (16 studies) or variational autoencoders (7 studies) to model patient-specific data [49]. These models have been applied to drug response prediction, treatment effect estimation, biomarker discovery, and patient stratification. For example, "Drug Response-VAE" architectures have been trained on cancer genomics to predict individual tumor sensitivity to drugs. Overall, generative AI has shown significant promise in enabling *precise treatment predictions and personalized therapeutic insights*. More broadly, supervised ML methods (random forests, boosting, deep networks) are used in pharmacogenomics to predict how genetic variants affect drug metabolism and efficacy. In oncology, AI helps match patients to targeted therapies by integrating mutation profiles and clinical features. Personalized dosing algorithms, powered by reinforcement learning or Bayesian optimization, dynamically adjust regimens in real time (for instance, in insulin pumps or chemotherapy). These AI-driven personalization tools can improve outcomes, though challenges remain in data diversity, model interpretability, and clinical validation [49].

1.4.3 AI in Pharmacovigilance

Post-marketing pharmacovigilance (drug safety monitoring) generates vast amounts of data from adverse events (AE) reports, literature, electronic health records, and social media. With AE reports growing *exponentially*, identifying "needles in the haystack" is a major challenge. AI and NLP methods are being applied to automate routine pharmacovigilance tasks. For example, ML algorithms can auto-code case reports (using MedDRA), de-duplicate reports, and triage serious vs. nonserious AEs without human review [50].

Natural language processing tools can scan unstructured sources (clinical notes, journals, patient forums, social media) to extract signals of drug-adverse event associations. In one survey, adopting AI tools was reported to greatly speed up case processing and analysis, saving time and effort compared to manual review. AI-driven signal detection algorithms can flag unusual patterns (e.g., clusters of symptoms) that warrant further investigation. By handling data entry and initial signal detection, AI augments the PV workforce, improving data quality and allowing human experts to focus on complex causality assessments. Nevertheless, full automation remains a goal; current limitations include data standardization issues, model interpretability, and regulatory concerns [50]. In summary, AI-based pharmacovigilance systems are already enhancing AE report processing and safety surveillance and are poised to further improve drug risk monitoring as methodologies mature.

References

1. Kandhare P, Kurlekar M, Deshpande T, Pawar A. A review on revolutionizing healthcare technologies with AI and ML applications in pharmaceutical sciences. Drugs Drug Candidates. 2025;4(1):9. https://doi.org/10.3390/ddc4010009.
2. Shanbhogue MH, Thirumaleshwar S, Tegginamath PK, Somareddy HK. Artificial intelligence in pharmaceutical field—a critical review. J Pharm Sci Res. 2021;18(10):1456–66. https://doi.org/10.2174/1567201818666210617100613.
3. Kulal N, Kumbhar N, Gaikwad O, Waghmode S, Adagale Y, Shinde N. Artificial intelligence in pharmaceutical sciences: an in-depth review from historical foundations to future innovations. Int J Sci R Tech. 2025;2(4):284–8. https://doi.org/10.5281/zenodo.15204206.
4. Vamathevan J, Clark D, Czodrowski P, et al. Applications of machine learning in drug discovery and development. Nat Rev Drug Discov. 2019;18:463–77. https://doi.org/10.1038/s41573-019-0024-5.
5. Chen H, Engkvist O, Wang Y, Olivecrona M, Blaschke T. The rise of deep learning in drug discovery. Drug Discov Today. 2018;23(6):1241–50. https://doi.org/10.1016/j.drudis.2018.01.039.
6. Goodfellow I, Bengio Y, Courville A. Deep learning. Cambridge, MA: MIT Press; 2016.
7. Mak KK, Pichika MR. Artificial intelligence in drug development: present status and future prospects. Drug Discov Today. 2019;24(3):773–80. https://doi.org/10.1016/j.drudis.2018.11.014.
8. Jumper J, Evans R, Pritzel A, et al. Highly accurate protein structure prediction with AlphaFold. Nature. 2021;596:583–9. https://doi.org/10.1038/s41586-021-03819-2.
9. Wadighare UA, Deshmukh SP. A review on artificial intelligence and machine learning used in pharmaceutical research. GSC Biol Pharm Sci. 2024;26(1):191–8. https://doi.org/10.30574/gscbps.2024.26.1.0446.
10. Javid S, Rahmanulla A, Ahmed MG, Sultana R, Kumar BRP. Machine learning & deep learning tools in pharmaceutical sciences. Comput Struct Biotechnol J. 2025;3(3):167–80. https://doi.org/10.1016/j.ipha.2024.11.003.
11. Kandhare P, Kurlekar M, Deshpande T, Pawar A. A review on revolutionizing healthcare technologies with AI and ML applications in pharmaceutical sciences. Drugs Drug Candidates. 2025;27:100375. https://doi.org/10.1016/j.medntd.2025.100375.
12. Shah M, Katkhade S, Gandhi S, Raut K, Haral R, Raut KJ, Kanase SS. A review on- artificial intelligence in pharmacy & applications of AI in pharmacy. Int J Pharm Sci. 2024;2(7):66–81. https://doi.org/10.5281/zenodo.12610382.

13. Mottaghi-Dastjerdi N, Soltany-Rezaee-Rad M. Advancements and applications of artificial intelligence in pharmaceutical sciences. Front Pharmacol. 2024;3(1):e150510. https://doi.org/10.5812/ijpr-150510.
14. Bajwa J, Munir U, Nori A, Williams B. Artificial intelligence in healthcare: transforming the practice of medicine. Future Healthc J. 2021;8:e188–94. https://doi.org/10.7861/fhj.2021-0095.
15. Xie Y, Zhai Y, Lu G. Evolution of artificial intelligence in healthcare: a 30-year bibliometric study. Front Med. 2025;11:1505692. https://doi.org/10.3389/fmed.2024.1505692.
16. Hirani R, Hirani R, Etienne M, et al. Artificial intelligence and healthcare: a journey through history, present innovations, and future possibilities. Life. 2024;14(5):557. https://doi.org/10.3390/life14050557.
17. Samajdar SS, Mukherjee S, Saboo B, et al. Artificial intelligence in healthcare: current trends and future directions. Curr Med Issues. 2025;23:53–60. https://doi.org/10.4103/cmi.cmi_93_24.
18. Faiyazuddin M, Rahman SJQ, Anand G, et al. The impact of artificial intelligence on healthcare: a comprehensive review of advancements in diagnostics, treatment, and operational efficiency. Health Sci Rep. 2025;8:e70312. https://doi.org/10.1002/hsr2.70312.
19. Topol EJ. High-performance medicine: the convergence of human and artificial intelligence. Nat Med. 2019;25:44–56. https://doi.org/10.1038/s41591-018-0300-7.
20. Yu K-H, Beam AL, Kohane IS. Artificial intelligence in healthcare. Nat Biomed Eng. 2018;2:719–31. https://doi.org/10.1038/s41551-018-0305-z.
21. Rajkomar A, Kohane I, Dean J. Machine learning in medicine. N Engl J Med. 2019;380:1347–58. https://doi.org/10.1056/nejmra1814259.
22. Obermeyer Z, Emanuel EJ. Predicting the future — big data, machine learning, and clinical medicine. N Engl J Med. 2016;375:1216–9. https://doi.org/10.1056/nejmp1606181.
23. Esteva A, Corrado G, Depristo M, et al. A guide to deep learning in healthcare. Nat Med. 2019;25:24–9. https://doi.org/10.1038/s41591-018-0316-z.
24. He J, Zhang K, Baxter SL, et al. The practical implementation of artificial intelligence technologies in medicine. Nat Med. 2019;25:30–6. https://doi.org/10.1038/s41591-018-0307-0.
25. Wang F, Casalino LP, Khullar D. Deep learning in medicine—promise, progress, and challenges. JAMA Intern Med. 2019;179(3):293–4. https://doi.org/10.1001/jamainternmed.2018.7117.
26. Davenport T, Kalakota R. The potential for artificial intelligence in healthcare. Future Healthc J. 2019;6:94–8. https://doi.org/10.7861/futurehosp.6-2-94.
27. Jiang F, Dong Y, Wang Y, et al. Artificial intelligence in healthcare: past, present and future. Stroke Vasc Neurol. 2017;2:230–43. https://doi.org/10.1136/svn-2017-000101.
28. Ebad SA, Alhashmi A, Amara M, et al. Artificial intelligence-based software as a Medical device (AI-SaMD): a systematic review. Healthcare (Basel, Switzerland). 2025;13:817. https://doi.org/10.3390/healthcare13070817.
29. Meskó B, Hetényi G, Győrffy Z. Will artificial intelligence solve the human resource crisis in healthcare? BMC Health Serv Res. 2018;18:545. https://doi.org/10.1186/s12913-018-3359-4.
30. Vasro. How AI is transforming drug discovery processes in 2025. Vasro 2025. https://vasro.de/en/impact-ai-drug-discovery-2025/
31. Fu C, Chen Q. The future of pharmaceuticals: artificial intelligence in drug discovery and development. J Pharm Anal. 2025;15:101248. https://doi.org/10.1016/j.jpha.2025.101248.
32. Ferreira FJN, Carneiro AS. AI-driven drug discovery: a comprehensive review. ACS Omega. 2025;10:23889–903. https://doi.org/10.1021/acsomega.5c00549.
33. Malheiro V, Santos B, Figueiras A, Mascarenhas-Melo F. The potential of artificial intelligence in pharmaceutical innovation: from drug discovery to clinical trials. Pharmaceuticals. 2025;18:788. https://doi.org/10.3390/ph18060788.
34. News-Medical. Why drug discovery needs robots and artificial intelligence. News-Medical 2025. https://www.news-medical.net/health/Why-Drug-Discovery-Needs-Robots-and-Artificial-Intelligence.aspx

35. Kadurin A, Aliper A, Nikolenko S, et al. druGAN: an advanced generative adversarial autoencoder model for de novo generation of new molecules with desired molecular properties in silico. Mol Pharm. 2017;14:3098–104. https://doi.org/10.1021/acs.molpharmaceut.7b00346.
36. Chen H, Engkvist O, Wang Y, et al. The rise of deep learning in drug discovery. Drug Discov Today. 2018;23:1241–50. https://doi.org/10.1016/j.drudis.2018.01.039.
37. Goh GB, Hodas NO, Vishnu A. Deep learning for computational chemistry. J Comput Chem. 2017;38:1291–307. https://doi.org/10.1002/jcc.24764.
38. Jarallah SJ, Almughem FA, Alhumaid NK, et al. Artificial intelligence revolution in drug discovery: a paradigm shift in pharmaceutical innovation. Int J Pharm. 2025;680:125789. https://doi.org/10.1016/j.ijpharm.2025.125789.
39. Zhavoronkov A, Soll R, Madge D, et al. Deep learning enables rapid identification of potent DDR1 kinase inhibitors. Nat Biotechnol. 2019;37:1038–40. https://doi.org/10.1038/s41587-019-0224-x.
40. Ching T, Do BT, Shrikumar A, et al. Opportunities and obstacles for deep learning in biology and medicine. J R Soc Interface. 2018;15:20170387. https://doi.org/10.1098/rsif.2017.0387.
41. Paul D, Sanap G, Shenoy S, et al. Artificial intelligence in drug discovery and development. Drug Discov Today. 2020;26:80–93. https://doi.org/10.1016/j.drudis.2020.10.010.
42. Ekins S, Lane TR, Klein JJ, et al. Exploiting machine learning for end-to-end drug discovery and development. Nat Mater. 2019;18:435–41. https://doi.org/10.1038/s41563-019-0338-z.
43. Walters WP, Barzilay R. Applications of deep learning in molecule generation and molecular property prediction. Acc Chem Res. 2020;54:263–70. https://doi.org/10.1021/acs.accounts.0c00699.
44. Lavecchia A. Deep learning in drug discovery: opportunities, challenges and future prospects. Drug Discov Today. 2019;24:2017–32. https://doi.org/10.1016/j.drudis.2019.07.006.
45. Schneider G. Automating drug discovery. Nat Rev Drug Discov. 2017;17:97–113. https://doi.org/10.1038/nrd.2017.232.
46. Vamathevan J, Clark D, Dunham I, et al. Applications of machine learning in drug discovery and development. Nat Rev Drug Discov. 2019;18:463–77. https://doi.org/10.1038/s41573-019-0024-5.
47. Qiu J, Li Y, Nguyen T, et al. From lab to clinic: how artificial intelligence (AI) is reshaping drug discovery and development. Pharmaceutics. 2025;18(7):981. https://doi.org/10.3390/pharmaceutics18070981.
48. Teodoro D, Naderi N, Yazdani A, Zhang B, Bornet A, et al. A scoping review of artificial intelligence applications in clinical trial risk assessment. NPJ Digit Med. 2025;8:486. https://doi.org/10.1038/s41746-025-01886-7.
49. Mishra A, Majumder A, Kommineni D, Joseph CA, Chowdhury T, Anumula SK. Role of generative artificial intelligence in personalized medicine: a systematic review. Cureus. 2025;17(4):e82310. https://doi.org/10.7759/cureus.82310.
50. Desai MK. Artificial intelligence in pharmacovigilance—opportunities and challenges. Perspect Clin Res. 2024;15(3):116–21. https://doi.org/10.4103/picr.picr_290_23.

2 AI in Early Drug Discovery

Contemporary drug development is notoriously slow, expensive, and failure prone. On average, it takes about 10–15 years and ~ $2.6 billion to bring a new drug to market, and fewer than 10% of candidates ultimately succeed. Most failures stem from inadequate target selection or unexpected safety issues. Against this backdrop, advanced computational methods have emerged to accelerate preclinical discovery. Modern machine learning and deep learning models can analyze vast, heterogeneous datasets—from genomics and proteomics to chemical libraries, uncovering patterns beyond traditional analyses. In recent reviews, experts emphasize that AI can "facilitate target identification with multi-omics data and network-based approaches" and likewise support virtual screening, de novo design, and lead optimization. These capabilities promise to reveal novel disease drivers, improve hit discovery, and optimize compound properties far more efficiently than classical methods [1]. It is estimated that the cost of discovering and developing a new drug is around USD 3 billion [2], with an approval rate close to 13% when considering all the compounds that reach clinical trials [3]. Novel compounds register an underwhelming success rate of ~66% in Phase I regarding tolerability and side effects, ~48% in Phase II concerning dosage and efficacy, and ~ 59% in Phase III regarding efficacy and toxicology [3].

2.1 Target Identification and Validation

Target identification is a key step in drug development [1]. AI has become a crucial tool offering the ability to analyze vast datasets, uncover hidden patterns, and propose novel therapeutic targets that may have been overlooked by traditional methods [4, 5]. AI-driven

K. Shaikh et al., *Artificial Intelligence in Drug Discovery and Development*,
Synthesis Lectures on Engineering, Science, and Technology,
https://doi.org/10.1007/978-3-032-10277-5_2

approaches not only streamline the target discovery process but also provide insights into complex biological networks that are key components of the oncogenic processes.

Early in the drug discovery process, *target identification* relies on interpreting complex biological data to find molecules that drive disease. Modern **multi-omics** approaches generate vast datasets—for example, sequencing patient genomes, transcriptomes, proteomes, and metabolomes—that capture complementary aspects of disease biology. Integrating these layers yields a far more complete picture than any single assay. In fact, recent reviews note that drug-target discovery has shifted toward multi-omics integration, effectively replacing older single-omics pipelines [6].

Artificial intelligence is ideally suited to this task: by sifting through genomic, transcriptomic, and proteomic data simultaneously, AI models can uncover subtle patterns and correlations that point to new targets. As one analysis explains, AI permits the analysis of "a large amount of data" that traditional statistics cannot manage [1]. The net result is a more systematic discovery of disease drivers and therapeutic targets.

- **Genomic analysis:** Whole-genome and exome sequencing identify genes that are frequently mutated or deleted in patients. Machine learning models can analyze these large datasets to prioritize genes that appear as recurrent drivers. For example, by integrating tumor genomic deletions with CRISPR loss-of-function screens, researchers found that cancers with an *MTAP* gene deletion are highly dependent on the enzyme PRMT5. This AI-driven insight highlighted PRMT5 as a synthetic-lethality target in those tumors [1]. These results show how AI can identify genes (such as PRMT5) that would be missed by less complex approaches.
- **Transcriptomic profiling**: High-throughput RNA sequencing, including single-cell RNA-seq, measures gene expression and splicing alterations in affected tissues. Millions of transcripts can be quickly scanned by machine learning to identify patterns linked to diseases. As an example, AI algorithms used to analyze a vast splicing database revealed aberrant transcriptomic signatures connected to pathology [7]. These models can rank genes whose dysregulation is strongly associated with the disease by correlating gene expression patterns with clinical outcomes. As a result, genes exhibiting the greatest variations in expression or unusual splicing events become high-priority targets.
- **Proteomics and metabolomics**: Quantitative proteomics identifies proteins whose abundance or modification changes in disease, while metabolomics measures shift in cellular pathways. AI tools can overlay proteomic and metabolomic data with other omic layers to pinpoint critical effectors. Recent studies have matched proteomic changes to genomic alterations to reveal new targets: for example, integration of proteomic profiles with genetic data uncovered previously unknown proteins central to disease mechanisms [6]. These AI-driven multi-omics analyses thus highlight proteins and pathways that might serve as therapeutic targets.
- **Integrated multi-omics analysis:** The greatest power comes from jointly analyzing all available data. By examining multiple omics layers in concert, AI models can

cross-validate results, for example, flagging a gene that is both mutated in the genome and overexpressed in the transcriptome. As Fan et al. observe, this integrative strategy "surpasses the information provided by single-omics analysis, enabling a more systematic study of the functionality and regulatory mechanisms of biological systems." In practice, multi-omics integration often constructs whole regulatory networks, revealing key molecular pathways and novel targets that emerge only when data are combined [6].

Classical drug discovery depends largely on HTS methods for screening enormous libraries of chemical compounds against the identified target in the discovery of novel chemical entities [8, 9]. To increase efficacy, these techniques were frequently coupled with structure-activity relationship (SAR) investigations, in which the biological activity of chemicals was correlated with their chemical structure [10]. The chosen chemicals may be chemically altered after these procedures to improve their characteristics, such as efficacy, selectivity, and pharmacokinetics, while simultaneously reducing toxicity and off-target effects. This procedure is known as lead optimization [1].

2.1.1 Network and Systems Biology Approaches

Diseases arise from complex networks of interacting genes and proteins, not isolated factors. AI excels at analyzing **biological networks** to find central nodes that serve as drug targets. For example, deep learning models (such as graph convolutional networks and recurrent neural nets) can be trained on known drug-target and protein–protein interaction networks to predict new target candidates [1]. These algorithms effectively identify "hub" genes or proteins whose perturbation would have a large impact on the network. In one approach, convolutional and recurrent neural networks learned from existing drug-target relationships and then predicted novel target associations beyond the training set [1].

- **Graph-based learning:** By representing genes and proteins as nodes in a graph and their interactions as edges, AI models can prioritize targets by network influence. For instance, a graph neural network can embed the human interactome into a low-dimensional space, scoring each gene by how central it is to disease pathways. These highlights topological "choke points" in disease networks that make attractive targets.
- **Convolutional and recurrent models:** CNNs and RNNs applied to interaction matrices have been used to forecast new drug-target edges. These models learn structural patterns from known interactions: for example, by feeding the neural net data on existing drug-compound and target relationships, the AI can extrapolate to predict which untested targets a compound might hit [1]. Such methods increase the hit rate of in silico target screening.
- **Generative and reinforcement learning:** AI can also create new therapeutic candidates targeting network hubs. Generative adversarial networks (GANs) and reinforcement learning systems design molecules with specific network-oriented objectives. For

instance, a GAN can propose compounds optimized to bind a particular protein network node, while a reinforcement learning model explores chemical space to improve target affinity. These AI-driven design processes tie directly back to target selection by focusing on the most promising nodes.

2.1.2 AI in Target Validation and Prioritization

After proposing targets, AI also aids *validation*, determining which targets are most likely to yield effective, safe drugs. ML models can simulate aspects of target validation before costly experiments. For example, supervised learning can predict the strength of binding between a candidate compound and a target (akin to virtual bioassays) [7]. By training on known binding data, these models triage targets by estimating which ones will be most tractable for drug binding.

AI also helps predict downstream effects of target modulation. By integrating biological networks and toxicity data, AI can estimate whether hitting a given target will achieve the desired effect and what side effects might occur. For instance, machine learning algorithms that analyze multi-omics perturbations can flag targets whose inhibition is predicted to restore normal cell function while warning of potential off-target toxicity. As one review notes, a major reason for drug failure is insufficient efficacy or safety, and AI approaches are being developed to predict these outcomes from molecular data [1]. In practice, models have been shown to reduce late-stage failures by filtering out high-risk targets early.

- **In silico binding validation:** AI can predict compound-target interactions en masse. By combining target structures (e.g., from AlphaFold) with virtual libraries, AI models can rapidly screen many target-ligand pairs to prioritize those with strongest predicted affinity [7]. This in silico step serves as a preliminary validation: if no compounds are predicted to bind a target well, it may be deprioritized before wet-lab assays.
- **Safety and efficacy prediction:** AI analyzes preclinical and omics data to estimate the therapeutic potential of a target. For example, by learning from historical drug data, ML tools can identify target features associated with toxicity or failure. Incorporating these predictions helps researchers focus on targets with the best risk/benefit profiles. According to Ocana et al., AI can "improve target identification and predict druggability," directly addressing the efficacy and safety challenges that most commonly derail drug candidates [1].
- **Prioritization via network modeling:** Complex network models can rank candidate targets by combining multiple criteria (disease relevance, druggability, network centrality). For instance, a recent AI framework applied to human interaction networks prioritized key Alzheimer's targets as candidates for drug repurposing [11]. Using such scoring, targets like *EGFR* and *RAC1* emerged on top as novel high-priority genes. This

illustrates how AI-enabled validation narrows a long list of hypotheses down to the most promising few.

- **Structural validation:** Finally, predicted protein structures themselves can validate target feasibility. The AlphaFold database, for example, provides 3D models that researchers can examine to confirm that a target has a suitable binding pocket. If the AI-generated structure shows a clear druggable groove, it supports moving forward; if not, the target might be deprioritized. In this way, structure-prediction AI becomes a tool for validating the "druggability" of new targets [7].

2.2 Virtual Screening and De Novo Drug Design

Early drug discovery relies heavily on virtual screening (VS) and de novo design, which allow for the exploration of large chemical spaces and the creation of novel ligands without the need for prior knowledge of known binders. Two complimentary behaviors emerged in recent years. First, ultra-large structure-based virtual screening is now possible due to an increase of commercially available chemical libraries, which today number in the billions, and computing advancements (cloud, GPUs, parallel clusters) [12, 13]. Second, both screening and design have been transformed by artificial intelligence and deep learning. Generative neural networks can suggest new molecules with desirable features, and machine learning can pre-filter or bias the selection of compounds in VS [14]. When combined, these developments allow for very large-scale silico searches and the production of custom molecules that are frequently experimentally confirmed iteratively. This chapter examines the most recent developments (about 2019–2025) in various fields, including deep learning-driven molecule production, AI-augmented screening, ultra-large VS platforms, and state-of-the-art screening methods. We provide examples and recent experimental triumphs throughout.

2.2.1 Ultra-Large Structure-Based Virtual Screening

Traditional structure-based VS docks virtual libraries into a protein binding site to identify likely binders. The availability of high-quality target structures (via X-ray crystallography, cryo-EM, or predicted by tools like AlphaFold) has dramatically expanded the reach of SBVS [13]. Indeed, with AlphaFold's 2021 breakthrough, "the structure of almost every protein known [has been] predicted and made freely available" (over 200 million entries in the AlphaFold database), meaning **SBVS can in principle be applied to most drug targets**. At the same time, ultra-large ready-to-dock libraries, e.g., Enamine's REAL space (tens of billions) or Zinc (billions), have emerged [12]. These enable broader exploration of chemical space but also pose severe computational challenges: docking even a few billion compounds by classical physics-based scoring is infeasible without optimizations.

To address this, specialized platforms and workflows have been developed. For example, **VirtualFlow** and other parallel docking frameworks distribute docking jobs across HPC clusters or cloud nodes, scaling to billions of compounds. In a recent demonstration, Zhou et al. constructed an open-source VS pipeline (OpenVS) combining Rosetta Ligand (with a custom force field) and deep learning guidance. Using 3000 CPUs and GPUs in parallel, they screened multi-billion libraries against two targets (human ubiquitin ligase KLHDC2 and NaV1.7 sodium channel). The entire campaign completed in under 7 days, yielding several new μM-active hits [12]. Such results underscore that multi-billion VS campaigns are now practicable: one group screened 11 billion compounds and discovered potent synthon-like ligands [12]. Likewise, Gorgulla et al. survey that ultra large VS (ULVS) has "enormous potential" and is already transforming early discovery [13]. In practice, these workflows often consist of iterative cycles: dock a random subset, train a model, focus on the highest-scoring region of chemical space, and repeat (often termed "active learning" docking) (a. overview of the deep learning guided virtual screening protocol; b. results of the area-under-curve (AUC) of the receiver operator characteristics (ROC) curve of the DUD benchmark, averaged over three independent runs (n = 3) and averaged over forty targets (n = 40); 95% confidence intervals are shown as error bars; c. mean ROC enrichments of the DUD benchmark at 0.5% (empty bar), 1% (patterned bar), and 2% (solid bar) false positive rates; results are averaged over three independent runs (n = 3) and averaged over 40 targets (n = 40); results of other methods are obtained from [15–17]; the same color scheme is used as in subpanel (b); d. CASF2016 docking power, the docking success rates of the top ten methods are shown; e. CASF2016 screening power, the top 1% enrichment factors with a 90% confidence interval of the top ten methods are shown; f. CASF2016 screening power, the success rates of the top ten methods are shown; results of other methods are obtained from [18]).

Key successes highlight this paradigm. For example, an AI-accelerated VS effort by Zhou et al. found five new binders (single-digit μM) from an initial screen of billions. These compounds were experimentally confirmed (one by X-ray crystallography) and subsequently extended through focused docking. Similarly, Luttens et al. (2025) combined docking with conformal prediction ML to screen ~10^{10} molecules across two GPCR targets, yielding a novel dual A2A/D2 agonist. These examples demonstrate that intelligent sampling (GPU-accelerated docking, parallelization, ML-guided selection) can overcome raw computational limits [12].

Despite these advances, some challenges remain. Highly accurate docking programs like Glide or GOLD have proven performance but are proprietary. Public tools (AutoDock Vina and its variants) remain popular but trade speed for some loss of accuracy. Moreover, even with parallelization, docking tens of billions of distinct 3D conformers is costly, motivating hybrid approaches. For instance, *virtual screening hierarchies* may combine ultra-fast 2D or pharmacophore filters before full 3D docking. Indeed, a recent high-profile approach (known as DOCK Blaster or Palladium) sequentially filters by ligand shape and fingerprint before refinement. In summary, current ULVS platforms employ multi-stage workflows on HPC: prepare huge libraries in ready-to-dock format, sample subsets or "synthon" spaces, run parallel docking (often on GPUs), and iterate with ML. The upshot is that lead identification, which once took months for a few thousand compounds, can now return μM hits in a matter of days from libraries of 10^9–10^11 molecules [12, 13].

A generative model is first pretrained on a large chemical database (e.g., ChEMBL) to learn valid molecular syntax. In an iterative optimization loop, molecules are sampled and evaluated by a property predictor; high-scoring molecules are stored in an "experience replay" buffer. The model is then refined via policy-gradient reinforcement learning, experience replay, and fine-tuning, using the buffer to bias generation toward active compounds. This cyclical process of generation, scoring, and retraining (illustrated here) is common in modern de novo design. The experimental training pipeline is shown in Fig. 2.1.

2.2.2 Machine Learning and AI in Virtual Screening

Machine learning (ML) now pervades virtual screening workflows. Instead of brute-force docking of every candidate, many pipelines use ML to **prioritize or predict docking**

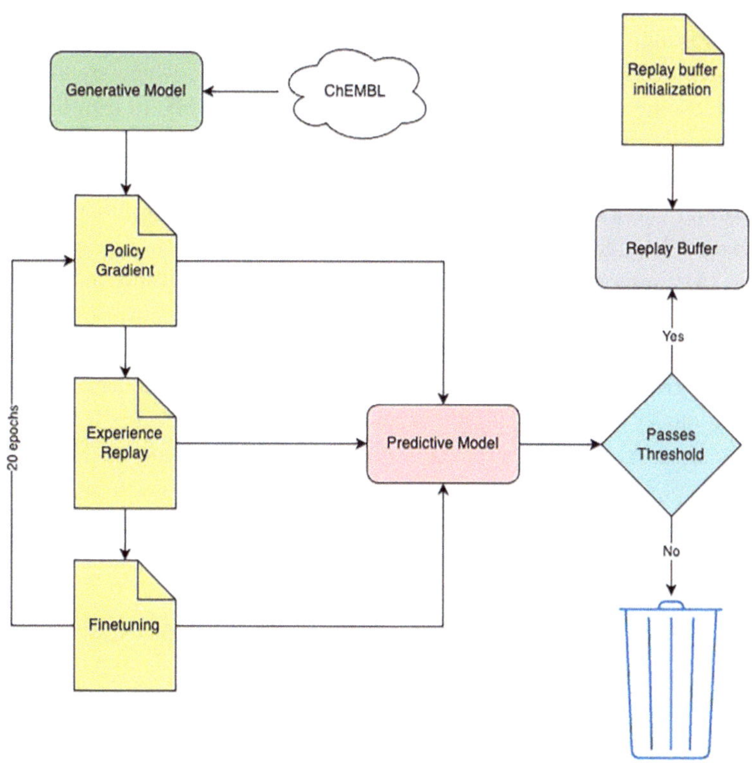

Fig. 2.1 Deep generative de novo design pipeline

scores. A prominent example is **Deep Docking (DD)** [14]. In the DD method, only a small random subset of a library is docked with a traditional scoring function, and a deep neural network is trained to predict docking scores for the rest [14]. Iterating this process (docking new high-scoring predictions to augment the training set) yields large accelerations. Gentile et al. report that DD can accelerate screening by 50–100× while achieving hundred- to thousand-fold enrichment of true hits. In practice, this has enabled docking of 10^9 compounds on modest clusters in 1–2 weeks, with little loss of potential hits. The DD code and protocols are freely available, exemplifying how ML and docking can co-operate.

Deep learning is also transforming the scoring phase of VS itself. Traditional scoring functions (empirical or force-field based) are being augmented or replaced by ML-based scoring. Convolutional 3D networks (e.g. AtomNet) can take a protein-ligand pose and estimate affinity. For example, the AtomNet architecture was tested in a "virtual HTS" on 318 diverse targets; it identified novel chemotypes for every target and, importantly, without known binders or exquisite structure quality [19]. Such results suggest that ML scoring can in some cases rival or exceed physical docking. However, hybrid experience suggests caution: Gao et al. (2024) note that when the binding site is well-known, physics-based docking still often outperforms blind ML predictions. In other words, ML is a powerful complement but not a complete replacement for docking yet [12].

Beyond scoring, AI can **pre-filter libraries** or design focused libraries. Generative models (discussed below) have been used to propose analogs, which are then filtered by docking/ML. Some groups use similarity or pharmacophore ML to trim libraries before docking. Others exploit **transfer learning**: a model pretrained on generic chemistry is fine-tuned on a small set of known actives (even synthetically unlabeled) to bias generation or scoring. These ligand-based filters (often ML regression or classification models) can cut an ultra-large library by orders of magnitude while retaining most hits [14].

Finally, "AI-augmented docking" frameworks are emerging. These include neural network potentials for fast pose sampling, generative adversarial networks to suggest conformers, and **equivariant neural networks** that predict binding geometries (e.g., DiffDock, TankBind). While such methods are typically faster, they are mainly suited to new binding modes rather than high-throughput VS where the pocket is known. Overall, the trend is clear: AI methods, especially deep learning, are being interwoven into each step of the VS pipeline. They guide which compounds to dock, how to predict their affinity, and even how to sample novel candidates, vastly accelerating screening of immense virtual libraries [12, 14].

2.2.3 Deep Learning for De Novo Molecular Design

While VS searches existing compounds, **de novo design** aims to *create* new molecules. Recent years have seen explosive growth in *generative* machine-learning models that propose entirely new structures. Deep generative models, including variational autoencoders

(VAEs), generative adversarial networks (GANs), autoregressive models (RNNs, transformers), and (most recently) diffusion networks are trained on large chemical datasets and learn to output valid SMILES or molecular graphs [20]. These models can be conditioned or optimized for target properties: for example, RNN-based models combined with reinforcement learning (RL) can maximize predicted binding affinity, physicochemical properties, or other objectives during generation.

A seminal example is the REINVENT framework, which uses an RNN trained on ChEMBL SMILES and fine-tunes it with policy-gradient RL. Korshunova et al. (2022) improved this paradigm by introducing experience replay and other tricks to balance exploration/exploitation. In one case study, they designed novel inhibitors of the EGFR kinase and *experimentally validated* their potency. Likewise, Zhavoronkov et al. (2019) famously used a generative tensor-RL model to design potent DDR1 kinase inhibitors, which were synthesized and confirmed in the lab [21]. These successes show that ML-driven design can reach real bioactive space.

More complex architectures are also emerging. Generative models can operate on 3D structures: for instance, Xu et al. (2024) developed a diffusion model that takes a protein pocket as input and generates matching ligand 3D structures. Diffusion networks—which iteratively "denoise" random input into molecular coordinates—have gained popularity for molecule generation. A cutting-edge example is the genotype-to-drug diffusion (G2D-Diff) model. Kim et al. (2025) trained G2D-Diff on cancer genotypes and drug response data. Given the genomic profile of, say, a triple-negative breast cancer, G2D-Diff generates diverse, drug-like compounds tailored to that condition [22]. In silico, it outperformed prior generative methods on diversity and property scores, and its attention module suggested relevant targets/pathways. This illustrates a new frontier: *personalized* generative design for precision medicine [23].

Other ML de novo approaches include graph-based VAEs (Jin et al., 2018) that assemble molecules fragment by fragment with guaranteed chemical validity and language models that treat SMILES as a "chemical language" (e.g., Chemformer, MolGPT). Generative models are increasingly incorporating domain knowledge: for example, the DeepBlock framework (Li et al., 2024) uses a rule-based block assembly inspired by DNA-encoded libraries [24]. Importantly, many of these models can optimize multiple objectives (binding, solubility, synthetic ease) simultaneously. For instance, multiobjective RL or Pareto optimization can tune generation to satisfy potency *and* ADMET constraints. These advances address a major limitation of early methods, which often produce unrealistic or insoluble molecules.

In practice, generative design often couples with VS in a loop: the ML model proposes novel candidates (e.g., via RL or conditional generation); these are then docked or experimentally tested; the feedback is used to further refine the model. For example, researchers might pretrain a VAE on ChEMBL and then fine-tune it with RL using a docking score or a pretrained binding-predictor as the reward. Over many epochs, the generator shifts toward outputting high-scoring ligands. The result can be entirely new scaffolds. Notably, these ML-generated leads can be explored by medicinal chemistry: computational hits are validated by synthesis and bioassay, as in the DDR1 and EGFR cases [25].

Finally, generative models are moving toward end-to-end AI platforms. Modern pipelines may integrate retrosynthetic prediction to ensure synthetic feasibility or use active learning to pick which virtual hits to synthesize. Some systems ("closed loop" molecular design) even automate the cycle, e.g., an AI suggests molecules, a lab robot synthesizes and tests them, and data is fed back to retrain the model. While such fully autonomous loops are nascent, they underscore the vision: AI-driven design and screening operating together to rapidly iterate on drug leads.

2.2.4 Emerging Screening Technologies and Future Directions

Complementing in silico advances, new experimental screening platforms are reshaping hit discovery. **DNA-encoded libraries (DELs)** exemplify this trend: by tagging each small molecule with a DNA barcode, researchers can screen trillions of compounds simultaneously against one or multiple targets in a single tube [20]. DEL selections require far less protein and compound than traditional high-throughput screening (HTS), yet sample orders of magnitude more structures. According to Peterson and Liu (2023), DEL technology has "matured into a widely used platform," delivering many clinical candidates. Its advantages—extreme library size, multiplexed assays, and efficient resource use—make DELs a powerful complement to VS and de novo approaches. In practice, computational methods are also applied to DELs (e.g., ML to analyze selection data and suggest next-generation libraries), merging the two fields.

Other cutting-edge methods include **fragment-based screening (FBS)** and **phenotypic screens**. FBS uses libraries of low-molecular-weight fragments (hundreds rather than millions of compounds) to probe binding sites via sensitive biophysical assays (NMR, X-ray crystallography, etc.). Hits are then elaborated into larger leads. AI is beginning to assist FBS by suggesting how to optimally merge or grow fragments [26]. Meanwhile, high-content phenotypic screens in cells or tissues, often using automated imaging ("cell painting"), generate rich multiparameter data. Machine learning can analyze these complex readouts to identify promising small molecules or predict targets. Although phenotypic screening lies somewhat outside classical VS, it represents a "cutting-edge" screening technology that benefits from data-driven analysis.

High-throughput screening itself is also evolving. Modern HTS systems use nanoliter-scale assays and robotics to test millions of compounds in days. Recent work suggests that well-trained neural networks might replace large-scale HTS in some cases: in a study of 318 targets, AtomNet predicted active compounds across diverse protein classes, without any physical screening. This points to a future where **computational screening substitutes for initial wet-lab screens** [19]. In practice, many organizations now use "synthetic-on-demand" libraries (trillions of make-on-command molecules) in combination with in silico triage: the top predictions are synthesized and tested, rather than testing every available compound. This hybrid virtual-experimental approach effectively blends VS with traditional screening.

On the computational side, ultra-large VS platforms and AI models open vast chemical spaces. On the experimental side, technologies like DELs and advanced HTS increase throughput and reduce costs. Crucially, these trends converge: AI models trained on experimental data (including DEL selections and phenotypic fingerprints) are now integral to the screening process, and virtual hits routinely move into automated synthesis and assay pipelines. Looking ahead, **integrated pipelines** combining ML-driven design, real-time bioassays, and active learning are anticipated. Such systems could continuously propose, test, and refine compounds, dramatically accelerating lead identification. As Gorgulla et al. note, the combination of ultra-large data and intelligent algorithms "is already starting to transform early-stage drug discovery" [13], heralding a future where virtual and experimental screening are tightly woven.

2.3 AI-Driven Chemical Space Exploration

Exploring chemical space—the conceptual universe of all possible small organic molecules—is a central challenge in early drug discovery. This space is astronomically large (often estimated on the order of 10^60 **drug-like** molecules), and naive enumeration or screening of this "vast, nearly infinite" space is infeasible [27]. Traditionally, chemists have defined chemical space via high-dimensional molecular descriptors (physicochemical properties, structural fingerprints, scaffolds, etc.), but navigating and visualizing this high-dimensional space requires powerful new approaches. Machine learning (ML) and deep learning offer such approaches: modern representation learning methods (e.g., graph neural networks (GNNs), variational autoencoders (VAEs), and transformers) can **encode molecules into continuous latent embeddings** that capture both local substructure and global features [27, 28]. These learned embeddings greatly improve the ability to search and interpolate in chemical space. In effect, AI-driven models learn a rich molecular "language" that goes beyond fixed expert-defined features, enabling smoother exploration and generation of new compounds, as shown in Fig. 2.2.

A common task is to **map** chemical space by projecting molecules into lower dimensions for visualization and analysis. For example, each molecule can be encoded by a high-dimensional fingerprint (e.g., ECFP) or a learned embedding, and then dimensionality reduction methods (PCA, t-SNE, UMAP, generative topographic mapping, etc.) are applied to visualize clusters of structurally or functionally similar compounds. Although these techniques have been used for years in chemoinformatics, AI enhances them: for instance, variational autoencoders (VAEs) learn smooth latent spaces such that similar molecules lie near each other in latent space [29]. These continuous latent spaces not only allow intuitive plots of chemical space but also enable **navigating** it by interpolation and sampling. In this way, AI-driven models create a "map" of chemical space where smooth movements correspond to chemically meaningful variations. Ultimately, molecular

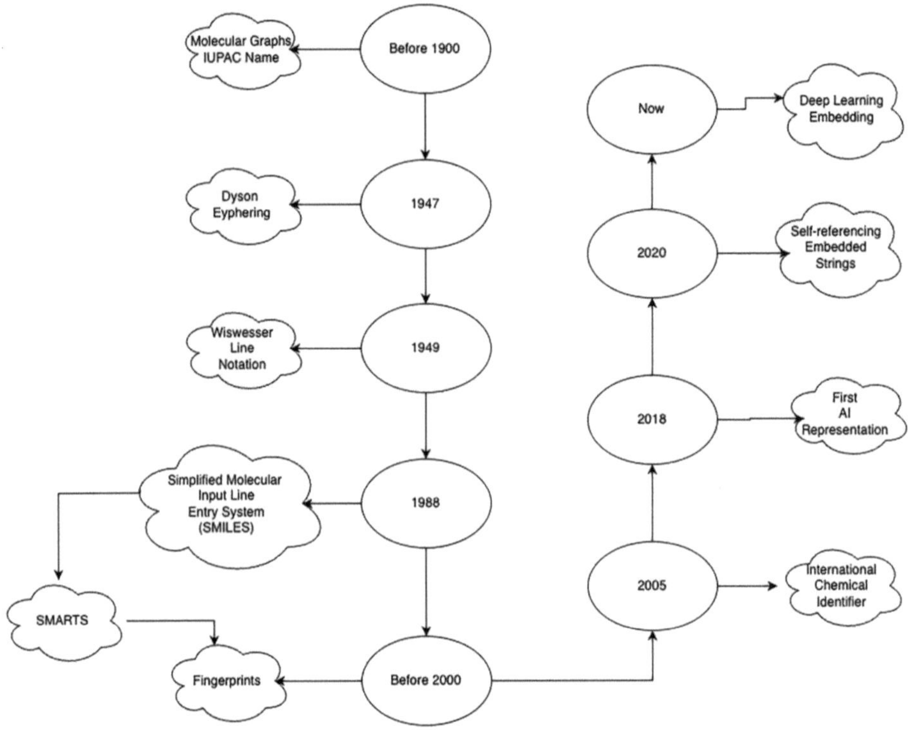

Fig. 2.2 Timeline of the initial proposals for various molecular representation methods

representation learning shifts the paradigm from rigid, predefined descriptors to flexible embeddings that better reflect molecular similarity and enable efficient search in enormous chemical libraries [30, 31].

2.3.1 Scaffold Hopping and Diversity in Chemical Libraries

Scaffold hopping discovering new molecular core structures ("scaffolds" or "chemotypes") that retain biological activity is a key strategy in lead optimization. Introduced by Schneider et al. in 1999, scaffold hopping aims to keep a compound's activity while replacing its central framework [32]. Representative strategies for scaffold hopping are shown in Fig. 2.3. Traditionally, scaffold hops were identified by medicinal chemists through intuition and substructure searches using fixed fingerprints or similarity measures [33]. However, these rule-based approaches struggle to traverse large chemical diversity: they often confine replacements to small modifications around known motifs.

Modern AI methods greatly expand scaffold-hopping capabilities by enabling **more flexible structure generation**. For example, recent generative reinforcement learning approaches train sequence models (e.g., SMILES-based LSTMs) to propose entirely new

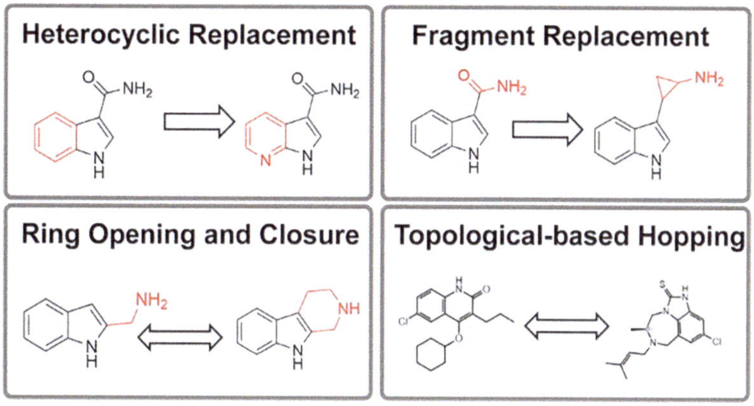

Fig. 2.3 Representative strategies for scaffold hopping

molecules. Rossen et al. (2025) developed *RuSH*, a reinforcement learning framework that generates whole molecules with high 3D-pharmacophore similarity to a reference compound but *low* common scaffold similarity [34]. In contrast to earlier methods that fixed a scaffold or linker, RuSH's **unconstrained** generation explores scaffold-diverse space: the model is rewarded for maximizing functional similarity while penalizing reuse of the original scaffold. In benchmark cases, RuSH outperformed prior approaches by systematically generating diverse new scaffolds that preserved key binding interactions. Such AI-driven scaffold hopping exemplifies how generative models can "jump" across chemical space, breaking free from the limitations of fixed-substructure rules and patent constraints [27, 34].

Modern AI methods greatly expand scaffold-hopping capabilities by enabling **more flexible structure generation**. For example, recent generative reinforcement learning approaches train sequence models (e.g., SMILES-based LSTMs) to propose entirely new molecules. Rossen et al. (2025) developed *RuSH*, a reinforcement learning framework that generates whole molecules with high 3D-pharmacophore similarity to a reference compound but *low* common scaffold similarity [34]. In contrast to earlier methods that fixed a scaffold or linker, RuSH's **unconstrained** generation explores scaffold-diverse space: the model is rewarded for maximizing functional similarity while penalizing reuse of the original scaffold. In benchmark cases, RuSH outperformed prior approaches by systematically generating diverse new scaffolds that preserved key binding interactions. Such AI-driven scaffold hopping exemplifies how generative models can "jump" across chemical space, breaking free from the limitations of fixed-substructure rules and patent constraints [27, 34].

Quantifying and ensuring **diversity** are another critical aspect of chemical space exploration. Compound libraries should cover broad regions of space to maximize the chance of finding novel hits. New diversity metrics have been developed to rigorously evaluate this coverage. For example, *sphere-exclusion* metrics (such as *SEDiv*) and the **#Circles** metric have been proposed to measure how well sets of molecules span chemical space [35]. In practice, one evaluates a model or library by how many diverse clusters or scaffolds it contains. Renz et al. (2024) demonstrated that many goal-directed generative models tend to produce clusters of very similar molecules. They proposed diversity-focused evaluations using the #Circles score to penalize such collapse. Their analysis showed that SMILES-based autoregressive models produced *significantly more diverse* molecules than graph-based models or genetic algorithms when optimized to a target. In other words, checking chemical diversity is now a standard way to validate generative exploration: a high-performance generator should not only achieve target properties but also maintain broad chemical variance [35].

2.3.2 Deep Learning Representations and Molecular Embeddings

Central to navigating chemical space is how molecules are represented in silico. Deep learning has introduced powerful new molecular embeddings that serve as coordinates in chemical space. One class of methods treats molecules as *sequences* (SMILES strings) and applies natural language processing techniques [36]. For instance, Jaeger et al.'s **Mol2Vec** treats molecular substructures (via the Morgan fingerprint algorithm) as "words" and entire molecules as "sentences," learning vector embeddings by a Word2Vec-like algorithm [27]. This unsupervised approach produces dense, information-rich vectors that capture substructure relationships and overcome sparsity issues of conventional fingerprints [37, 38]. BERT-based models (transformer encoders) have also been adapted: *Mol-BERT*, *MTL-BERT*, and *MolRoPE-BERT* are pretrained on massive SMILES corpora using masked language modeling. These models learn contextual embeddings where each token's vector reflects its molecular environment. Li et al. showed that Mol-BERT's embeddings, fine-tuned for property prediction, outperform traditional graph-based features, because they capture subtle atom-substructure contexts [39]. Such language-model embeddings encapsulate rich chemical semantics, enabling downstream tasks like property prediction or scaffold ranking to benefit from pre-learned chemical knowledge [27].

Another powerful approach is **graph neural networks (GNNs)**, which directly encode molecules as graphs (atoms = nodes; bonds = edges). GNNs learn to propagate information through the molecular graph, capturing both local and global structural patterns. This is highly effective for chemical tasks because it mirrors the physical structure of molecules: similar subgraphs lead to similar embeddings. For example, the attentive FP model aggregates atomic environments through attention mechanisms, and GROVER (a GNN + Transformer hybrid) uses large-scale self-supervised pretraining on unlabeled molecular graphs [27]. In general, GNNs automatically learn descriptors of rings, functional groups, and graph topology, yielding embeddings that correlate directly with chemical properties. These graph-based embeddings are ideally suited for molecular generation and property prediction: a single vector can summarize a molecule's structure in a way that ML models readily exploit.

Self-supervised learning further enriches these embeddings. Models pretrained on unlabeled molecules (using tasks like random atom masking or contrastive graph learning) produce latent vectors that capture nuanced chemical information beyond any single descriptor [39, 40]. For instance, GROVER's masked graph prediction and GraphMVP's 2D/3D alignment learning have shown that embedding pretraining yields more expressive and transferable chemical representations. Such unsupervised strategies allow chemical models to learn from vast amounts of data without requiring property labels. The resulting latent spaces place similar molecules nearby and often organize compounds by scaffold or property trends, making the space easier to search or cluster. In summary, deep representation learning has revolutionized chemical space mapping: by turning discrete molecules into smooth, high-dimensional vectors, AI can measure distances, interpolate, and optimize directly in chemical space [41].

2.3.3 Generative Models and Structure-Property Landscape Modeling

Beyond analyzing existing compounds, AI enables the **de novo generation** of novel molecules to populate chemical space. Generative models such as VAEs, generative adversarial networks (GANs), and diffusion models have emerged as potent tools for this purpose. VAEs encode molecules into continuous latent vectors and decode random samples from this space back into molecules [29]. The smooth latent manifold of a VAE ensures that nearby points decode to chemically similar and valid structures. By sampling from or optimizing in this latent space, one can efficiently traverse unexplored regions of chemical space. As one review notes, "Generative models… allow researchers to explore vast chemical spaces with unprecedented depth and efficiency" [30, 31]. Variational autoencoders and their variants (deep VAEs, InfoVAEs, GraphVAEs) have been successfully applied to molecular design, often trained together with property predictors to bias generation toward desired characteristics. Likewise, diffusion models (which progressively add and remove noise to generate structures) and GANs (which pit a molecular generator against a discriminator) offer complementary generative paradigms, each capable of proposing entirely new scaffolds that were not in any training set [28].

Critically, these generative frameworks support **structure-property landscape modeling** by coupling generation with property evaluation. One strategy is *property-guided generation*, where the model is steered to satisfy targets. For example, the *GaUDI* framework uses an equivariant GNN to predict a molecule's properties, then a diffusion model to sample structures that optimize those properties. More generally, reinforcement learning (RL) and Bayesian optimization have been integrated with generative models to perform goal-directed search in chemical space. RL agents (e.g., MolDQN) iteratively modify molecules and receive rewards based on properties like activity, drug-likeness, or similarity to a reference. Balancing exploration versus exploitation is a key challenge; advanced approaches use uncertainty-aware networks or memory-based filters to encourage diversity while optimizing property scores. Graph convolutional policy networks (GCPN) are another RL example, where the agent constructs molecules atom-by-atom to maximize a composite reward. Overall, AI-driven generation turns chemical space exploration into an adaptive search problem: agents learn to propose molecules that both inhabit new regions of the space and improve predicted properties.

Unsupervised generative models also expose the intrinsic **landscape** of chemical space. By training on large molecular datasets without labels, models like VAEs or autoencoders implicitly learn the global structure-property relationships. Clusters in the latent space often correspond to families of scaffolds or activity classes, revealing the underlying topology of chemical diversity. Conversely, problematic "activity cliffs" (small structural changes causing large property jumps) can be identified as discontinuities in the landscape; recent methods even explicitly model these cliffs during generation to improve robustness. In practice, one can sample from a VAE latent region known to contain active compounds to generate analogs or perform local interpolation between high-scoring points to chart smooth paths of SAR change. In this way, structure-property landscape modeling becomes tractable: AI offers a continuous view of the chemical universe, where optimization algorithms can navigate toward optimal compounds. The synergy of unsupervised learning and generative sampling thus provides unprecedented coverage of chemical space, expanding the search beyond what traditional enumeration or screening could achieve [29].

AI-driven chemical space exploration unites theoretical mapping and practical design. Deep embeddings turn molecules into points in a learned high-dimensional space; diversity metrics and scaffold-aware scoring guide searches for novel structures [34, 35]; and generative models actively propose new compounds optimized for target properties [28]. Recent literature demonstrates that these AI techniques can outperform classical methods in scaffold hopping, generate more chemically diverse libraries, and effectively model complex structure-activity landscapes. As research progresses, we expect further integration of these approaches (e.g., multiobjective optimization, active learning) and more open-source resources for traversing chemical space. Together, these advances are rapidly extending the frontier of early drug discovery into previously unreachable regions of chemical space, potentially accelerating the identification of novel drug candidates with improved efficacy and safety.

2.4 Case Studies of Successful Early Discoveries

Recognizing crucial signals ahead of others is frequently the source of early advancements in science and technology. Methodical early discovery has produced paradigm-shifting outcomes across a wide range of sectors, including physics, medicine, and public health. Drawing on peer-reviewed reports and expert accounts, the following case studies demonstrate how proactive identification or analysis led to significant accomplishments.

2.4.1 Gravitational Waves: LIGO'S Pioneering Discovery

For the first time, gravitational waves, which are ripples in spacetime, were detected by the two LIGO detectors in September 2015 [42]. Two enormous black holes spiraling inward and colliding produced this revolutionary signal, which Einstein's theory of general relativity has long predicted. The first direct observation of gravitational waves, which perfectly matched theoretical models, was made by LIGO, who proudly announced that it "confirms a major prediction of Albert Einstein's 1915 general theory of relativity and opens an unprecedented new window onto the cosmos" [42]. The measure was recognized as a watershed achievement in physicsui.adsabs.harvard.edu and had an extremely high statistical significance in practical terms (false alarm rate of less than 1 in 200,000 years).

The early success of LIGO had a quick and widespread effect. Scientists established gravitational wave astronomy by discovering spacetime ripples, which also supported Einstein's hundred-year-old theory. According to a Physical Review Letters article, the merger of two black holes, one with around 36 solar masses and the other with 29 solar masses, occurred 1.3 billion years ago. Since then, it has made it possible to find hundreds of additional signals from black holes and neutron stars, and it also won the LIGO founders the 2017 Nobel Prize. This achievement, according to Caltech's statement, "accomplishes an ambitious goal set out over 5 decades ago" and ushers in a new age of monitoring cosmic phenomena that were previously unseen by conventional telescopes. In conclusion, the LIGO experiment demonstrates how careful, high-accuracy monitoring can identify unusual signals in their early stages and revolutionize our knowledge of the cosmos [42].

2.4.2 Mammography Screening: Reducing Cancer Mortality

Medical screening is another area where early detection has saved many lives. By detecting malignancies at an earlier, more curable stage, large-scale breast cancer screening programs have significantly reduced mortality. For example, data from the US Surveillance, Epidemiology, and End Results (SEER) program shows that the mortality rate for breast cancer in the United States has decreased by about 40% since the 1980s, when mammography became widely used [43]. From a practical standpoint, women who get mammograms on a regular basis are far less likely to die from cancer than those who do not. According to a large Swedish study, women who received regular screenings had a 41% decreased chance of dying from breast cancer within 10 years of their diagnosis. The same study also found that for women in screening programs, there was a 25% reduction in cases diagnosed at an advanced stage [44].

Broader studies corroborate these conclusions. According to the American College of Radiology, women who are screened have around half the risk of dying from breast cancer as their unscreened counterparts. Mammography enables early detection, which means that malignancies are discovered at a smaller, less likely to have spread stage, allowing for less invasive therapy and a better prognosis. The advantages of screening are seen "independent of treatment regimen," as Dr. László Tabár, a pioneer in Swedish screening, points out, emphasizing that the decline in mortality is brought about by screening alone. Dozens of nations have used this data to establish national mammography programs, and several follow-up trials have supported the conclusion that early breast cancer detection results in lives saved. This example highlights how well-organized, universal screening can make use of early detection to achieve remarkable success in disease management [43, 44].

2.4.3 Protein Folding: The AlphaFold Revolution

Protein structure prediction was a grand challenge for over 50 years: knowing a protein's folded 3D shape from its sequence would unlock biological insight and drug design. In 2020, the AI program AlphaFold achieved what experimental methods could only do with great effort. In the blind Critical Assessment of Protein Structure Prediction (CASP14), AlphaFold produced atomic-level accuracy predictions for most targets, far outperforming all competitors [45]. Specifically, the latest AlphaFold achieved a median error of only ~1.6 Å (angstroms) on these tests, a level comparable to experimental structures. Researchers hailed the result as "the first computational method that can regularly predict protein structures with atomic accuracy even in cases in which no similar structure is known." Nobel Laureate Venki Ramakrishnan described this as "a stunning advance on the protein-folding problem occurring decades before many people in the field would have predicted" [46].

AlphaFold's early success has already catalyzed downstream discoveries. Its accurate predictions have been made freely available for vast numbers of proteins, essentially solving structures that would otherwise take years of lab work. Biologists now routinely use these models to infer function and guide experiments. As the DeepMind team summarized, their neural-network model "demonstrated accuracy competitive with experimental structures in a majority of cases and greatly outperforming other methods" [45]. This breakthrough has accelerated drug discovery, enzyme engineering, and basic research. In essence, a complex scientific question (folding a protein) has been *discovered* computationally with reliability; researchers no longer wait for laborious crystallography for many targets. The AlphaFold story highlights how a data-driven approach can achieve an early breakthrough, leapfrogging traditional timelines in molecular biology.

2.4.4 Wastewater Surveillance: An Early Warning for Outbreaks

In public health, innovative surveillance methods have enabled detection of disease trends before clinical diagnoses rise. Wastewater-based epidemiology is one such success. By testing community sewage for viral genetic material, officials can monitor infections in the population at large. Experts note that wastewater surveillance "has proven to be successful in describing epidemiological trends by identifying and quantifying the virus RNA in wastewater samples" [47, 48]. Crucially, increases in viral load in sewage often precede confirmed case counts. For example, a 2024 study in Caracas (Venezuela) found that SARS-CoV-2 RNA concentrations in sewer systems foreshadowed COVID-19 case spikes by roughly a week. The authors concluded that this method "can serve as an early warning system for SARS-CoV-2 outbreaks" and complements traditional surveillance, especially in areas with underreporting [49].

Broad implementation of wastewater monitoring has proven its value. By late 2022, the US Centers for Disease Control and Prevention (CDC) had linked over 1200 testing sites nationwide in a wastewater surveillance network [50]. This system now covers wastewater systems serving over 130 million people, and CDC highlights it as "providing an important early warning signal of increasing infections." Indeed, genomic sequencing of sewage samples has even signaled the arrival of new variants. For instance, CDC reported finding Omicron-specific mutations in wastewater in November 2021 before clinical cases were detected in those communities. These examples show how detecting pathogens in sewage translates into early outbreak discovery and timely response. When properly implemented, this approach allows public health teams to act days before a surge becomes evident in clinics or hospitals [48].

Each case above draws on rigorous research and field data to demonstrate that early discovery, be it of cosmic waves, a looming infection, or a molecular structure, can yield profound benefits. By investing in the capability to detect subtle signals or model outcomes ahead of traditional means, scientists and societies have achieved results that would have been impossible with reactive approaches alone [42, 48]. These examples collectively reinforce the value of vigilant monitoring and innovative analytics in realizing timely, life-changing discoveries.

References

1. Ocana A, Pandiella A, Privat C, et al. Integrating artificial intelligence in drug discovery and early drug development: a transformative approach. Biomark Res. 2025;13:45. https://doi.org/10.1186/s40364-025-00758-2.
2. Wouters OJ, McKee M, Luyten J. Estimated research and development investment needed to bring a new medicine to market, 2009-2018. JAMA. 2020;323(9):844–53.
3. Wong CH, Siah KW, Lo AW. Estimation of clinical trial success rates and related parameters. Biostatistics. 2019;20(2):273–86.
4. Rudolph J, Settleman J, Malek S. Emerging trends in cancer drug discovery—from drugging the undruggable to overcoming resistance. Cancer Discov. 2021;11:815–21.
5. Menyhárt O, Győrffy B. Multi-omics approaches in cancer research with applications in tumor subtyping, prognosis, and diagnosis. Comput Struct Biotechnol J. 2021;19:949–60.
6. Du P, Fan R, Zhang N, Wu C, Zhang Y. Advances in integrated multi-omics analysis for drug-target identification. Biomolecules. 2024;14(6):692. https://doi.org/10.3390/biom14060692.
7. Colwell NA. Harnessing artificial intelligence in drug discovery and development. ACCC Buzz [blog] 20 Dec 2024. https://www.accc-cancer.org/acccbuzz/blog-post-template/

accc-buzz/2024/12/20/harnessing-artificial-intelligence-in-drug-discovery-and-development. Accessed 4 Aug 2025.

8. Li R, et al. Comparative optimization of combinatorial CRISPR screens. Nat Commun. 2022;13:2469.
9. Macarron R, et al. Impact of high-throughput screening in biomedical research. Nat Rev Drug Discov. 2011;10:188–95.
10. Liew SK, Malagobadan S, Arshad NM, Nagoor NH. A review of the Structure–Activity relationship of natural and synthetic antimetastatic compounds. Biomolecules. 2020;10:138.
11. Tsuji S, Hase T, Yachie-Kinoshita A, et al. Artificial intelligence-based computational framework for drug-target prioritization and inference of novel repositionable drugs for Alzheimer's disease. Alzheimers Res Ther. 2021;13:92. https://doi.org/10.1186/s13195-021-00826-3.
12. Zhou G, Rusnac DV, Park H, et al. An artificial intelligence accelerated virtual screening platform for drug discovery. Nat Commun. 2024;15:7761. https://doi.org/10.1038/s41467-024-52061-7.
13. Gorgulla C. Recent developments in structure-based virtual screening approaches. Annu Rev Pharmacol Toxicol. 2024;64:477–502. https://doi.org/10.1146/annurev-pharmtox-021023-095711.
14. Gentile F, Yaacoub JC, Gleave J, et al. Artificial intelligence–enabled virtual screening of ultra-large chemical libraries with deep docking. Nat Protoc. 2022;17:672–97. https://doi.org/10.1038/s41596-021-00659-2.
15. Cross JB, et al. Comparison of several molecular docking programs: pose prediction and virtual screening accuracy. J Chem Inf Model. 2009;49:1455–74.
16. Arciniega M, Lange OF. Improvement of virtual screening results by docking data feature analysis. J Chem Inf Model. 2014;54:1401–11.
17. Pereira JC, Caffarena ER, dos Santos CN. Boosting docking-based virtual screening with deep learning. J Chem Inf Model. 2016;56:2495–506.
18. Shen C, et al. Boosting protein–ligand binding pose prediction and virtual screening based on residue–atom distance likelihood potential and graph transformer. J Med Chem. 2022;65:10691–706.
19. The Atomwise AIMS Program. AI is a viable alternative to high throughput screening: a 318-target study. Sci Rep. 2024;14:7526. https://doi.org/10.1038/s41598-024-54655-z.
20. Peterson AA, Liu DR. Small-molecule discovery through DNA-encoded libraries. Nat Rev Drug Discov. 2023;22:699–722. https://doi.org/10.1038/s41573-023-00713-6.
21. Zhavoronkov A, et al. Deep learning enables rapid identification of potent DDR1 kinase inhibitors. Nat Biotechnol. 2019;37:1038–40. https://doi.org/10.1038/s41587-019-0224-x.
22. Kim H, Bae B, Park M, et al. A genotype-to-drug diffusion model for generation of tailored anti-cancer small molecules. Nat Commun. 2025;16:5628. https://doi.org/10.1038/s41467-025-60763-9.
23. Ho J, Jain A, Abbeel P. Denoising diffusion probabilistic models. Adv Neural Inf Process Syst. 2020;33:6840–51.
24. Li P, Zhang K, Liu T, et al. A deep learning approach for rational ligand generation with toxicity control via reactive building blocks. Nat Comput Sci. 2024;4:851–64. https://doi.org/10.1038/s43588-024-00718-0.
25. Korshunova M, Huang N, Capuzzi S, et al. Generative and reinforcement learning approaches for the automated de novo design of bioactive compounds. Commun Chem. 2022;5:129. https://doi.org/10.1038/s42004-022-00733-0.
26. Bon M, Bilsland A, Bower J, McAulay K. Fragment-based drug discovery—the importance of high-quality molecule libraries. Mol Oncol. 2022;16(21):3761–77. https://doi.org/10.1002/1878-0261.13277.

27. Wang S, Zhang R, Li X, et al. Recent advances in molecular representation methods and their applications in scaffold hopping. NPJ Drug Discov. 2025;2:14. https://doi.org/10.1038/s44386-025-00017-2.
28. Khater T, Alkhatib SA, AlShehhi A, et al. Generative artificial intelligence based models optimization towards molecule design enhancement. J Cheminform. 2025;17:116. https://doi.org/10.1186/s13321-025-01059-4.
29. Kingma DP, Welling M. An introduction to variational autoencoders. Found trends® Mach Learn. 2019;12(4):307–92. https://doi.org/10.1561/2200000056.
30. Luo Y, Zhang T, Sun H, Lin X, Liu Y, Wu Z, Li Z. Text-guided small molecule generation via diffusion model. iScience. 2024;27(11):110992. https://doi.org/10.1016/j.isci.2024.110992.
31. Datta J, Datta D, Nadimpally A, Koratkar N. Generative AI for discovering porous oxide materials for next-generation energy storage. arXiv 2024. https://doi.org/10.4855/arXiv.2410.06433
32. Schneider G, Neidhart W, Giller T, Schmid G. "Scaffold-hopping" by topological pharmacophore search: a contribution to virtual screening. Angew Chem Int Ed. 1999;38:2894–6.
33. Sun HM, Tawa G, Wallqvist A. Classification of scaffold-hopping approaches. Drug Discov Today. 2012;17:310–24.
34. Rossen L, Sirockin F, Schneider N, Grisoni F. Scaffold hopping with generative reinforcement learning. J Chem Inf Model. 2025;65(13):6513–25. https://doi.org/10.1021/acs.jcim.5c00029.
35. Renz P, Luukkonen S, Klambauer G. Diverse hits in de novo molecule design: diversity-based comparison of goal-directed generators. J Chem Inf Model. 2024;64(15):5756–61. https://doi.org/10.1021/acs.jcim.4c00519.
36. Shao JS, Jia QF, Chen X, Hao YJ, Wang L. Molecular fragmentation as a crucial step in the AI-based drug development pathway. Commun Chem. 2024;7:20. https://doi.org/10.1038/s42004-024-01017-0.
37. Jaeger S, Fulle S, Turk S. Mol2vec: unsupervised machine learning approach with chemical intuition. J Chem Inf Model. 2018;58(1):27–35. https://doi.org/10.1021/acs.jcim.7b00616.
38. Mikolov T, Chen K, Corrado GS, Dean J. Efficient estimation of word representations in vector space. In: International Conference on Learning Representations (ICLR); 2013.
39. Li Q, He Y, Pan JB. CrossFuse-XGBoost: accurate prediction of the maximum recommended daily dose through multi-feature fusion, cross-validation screening and extreme gradient boosting. Brief Bioinform. 2024;25:bbad511.
40. Ji ZW, Shi RH, Lu JR, Li F, Yang Y. ReLMole: molecular representation learning based on two-level graph similarities. J Chem Inf Model. 2022;62(21):5361–72.
41. Li Y, Zhang C, Wang Q, Zhao Y, Liu Z, Yang Y, et al. An adaptive graph learning method for automated molecular interactions and properties predictions. Nat Mach Intell. 2022;4:645–51.
42. LIGO Caltech. Gravitational waves detected 100 years after Einstein's prediction: LIGO opens new window on the universe with observation of gravitational waves from colliding black holes. News release, 11 Feb 2016. https://www.ligo.caltech.edu/news/ligo20160211. Accessed 4 Aug 2025.
43. American College of Radiology. ACR statement on Harris opinion editorial. News release, 5 Feb 2024. https://www.acr.org/News-and-Publications/Media-Center/2024/ACR-Statement-on-Annals-of-Internal-Medicine-Harris-Opinion-Editorial. Accessed 4 Aug 2025.
44. Duffy SW, Tabár L, Yen AM-F, et al. Mammography screening reduces rates of advanced and fatal breast cancers: results in 549,091 women. Cancer. 2020;126(13):2971–9. https://doi.org/10.1002/cncr.32859.
45. Moult J, Fidelis K, Kryshtafovych A, Schwede T, Topf M. Critical assessment of techniques for protein structure prediction, fourteenth round. CASP 14 Abstract Book. 2020. https://www.predictioncenter.org/casp14/doc/CASP14_Abstracts.pdf

46. The AlphaFold Team. AlphaFold: a solution to a 50-year-old grand challenge in biology. DeepMind blog 30 Nov 2020. https://deepmind.google/discover/blog/alphafold-a-solution-to-a-50-year-old-grand-challenge-in-biology/. Accessed 4 Aug 2025.
47. Ahmed W, Angel N, Edson J, et al. First confirmed detection of SARS-CoV-2 in untreated wastewater in Australia: a proof of concept for the wastewater surveillance of COVID-19 in the community. Sci Total Environ. 2020;728:138764. https://doi.org/10.1016/j.scitotenv.2020.138764.
48. Nauta M, McManus O, Træholt Franck K, Lindberg Marving E, Dam Rasmussen L, Raith Richter S, Ethelberg S. Early detection of local SARS-CoV-2 outbreaks by wastewater surveillance: a feasibility study. Epidemiol Infect. 2023;151:e28. https://doi.org/10.1017/S0950268823000146.
49. Bastardo-Méndez M, Rangel HR, Pujol FH, et al. Detection of SARS-CoV-2 in wastewater as an earlier predictor of COVID-19 epidemic peaks in Venezuela. Sci Rep. 2024;14:27294. https://doi.org/10.1038/s41598-024-78982-3.
50. Centers for Disease Control and Prevention. Wastewater Surveillance: a New Frontier for Public Health. https://www.cdc.gov/advanced-molecular-detection/php/success-stories/wastewater-surveillance.html. Published April 15, 2024. Accessed 11 Aug 11 2025.

AI for Preclinical and Translational Research

3

3.1 Introduction to AI in Preclinical and Translational Research

Preclinical as well as translational research belongs to the initial steps of drug development and aims to translate scientific findings into potential therapeutic concepts. However, these phases are usually lengthy and resource-intensive and have high failure rates. A significant third bottleneck impeding achievement is the gap between the results of preclinical experimentation and their application to human treatment; even though R&D in the pharmaceutical industry amounts to billions of dollars, the proportion of successful translations from animal experiments to human treatment is disturbingly low. Over 90% of drug proposals fail during clinical development, and the average cost to bring a new medicine to market is estimated to be over $2.6 billion [1]. With the potential to enhance decision-making, lower expenses, and shorten timelines throughout the biomedical innovation pipeline, artificial intelligence (AI) has become a disruptive force in this regard.

3.1.1 The Evolving Role of AI

Artificial intelligence refers to a group of computational techniques that allow machines to recognize patterns in data and make decisions or predictions, such as machine learning (ML), deep learning (DL), and natural language processing (NLP). These technologies have been extremely helpful in biomedical research for tasks including image processing, high-throughput screening, molecular property prediction, and omics data integration. An overview of AI-driven multi-omics integration is shown in Fig. 3.1 [2]. Unprecedented potential to extract insights from the large and intricate datasets that define contemporary life sciences have been made possible by the confluence of AI with big data, cloud computing, and high-performance GPUs [3]. In preclinical research, AI is increasingly used to:

K. Shaikh et al., *Artificial Intelligence in Drug Discovery and Development*,
Synthesis Lectures on Engineering, Science, and Technology,
https://doi.org/10.1007/978-3-032-10277-5_3

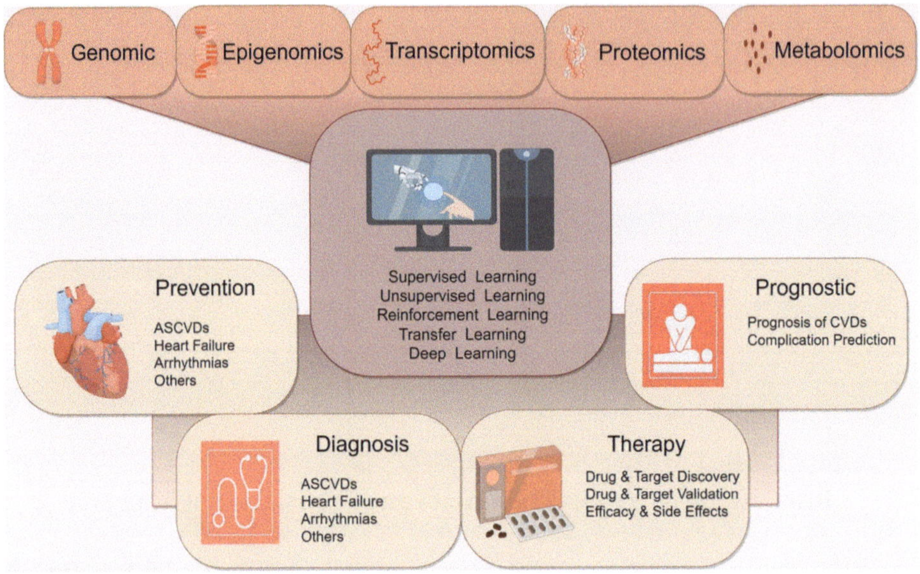

Fig. 3.1 An overview of AI-driven multi-omics integration

- Predict compound toxicity and pharmacokinetics.
- Identify novel disease biomarkers.
- Analyze and integrate multi-omics datasets.
- Automate high-content screening and phenotypic assays.
- Support hypothesis generation and drug repurpose.

These features not only increase preclinical models' predictive ability but also provide a pathway to translational research, where results are modified for use in clinical settings. For instance, by linking molecular profiles to therapeutic outcomes, AI can assist in determining which patient subgroups are most likely to benefit from a new medication [4]. Figure 3.2 shows schematic of the ML pipeline in multi-omics studies [2].

3.1.2 Data-Driven Vs. Hypothesis-Driven Research

Traditional biomedical research has mostly been hypothesis-driven, with scientists designing trials to verify certain mechanistic theories. Even though this approach has yielded important results, human bias and the study's scope invariably limit it. Conversely, AI is particularly good at data-driven discovery, which identifies patterns without the use of assumptions. When working with high-dimensional data, like imaging, proteomics, and genomes, this is extremely beneficial (see Fig. 3.3). For instance, unsupervised learning algorithms may classify patient data based on genetic markers, identifying novel illness categories that may respond differently to treatment. Similarly, by learning from previous

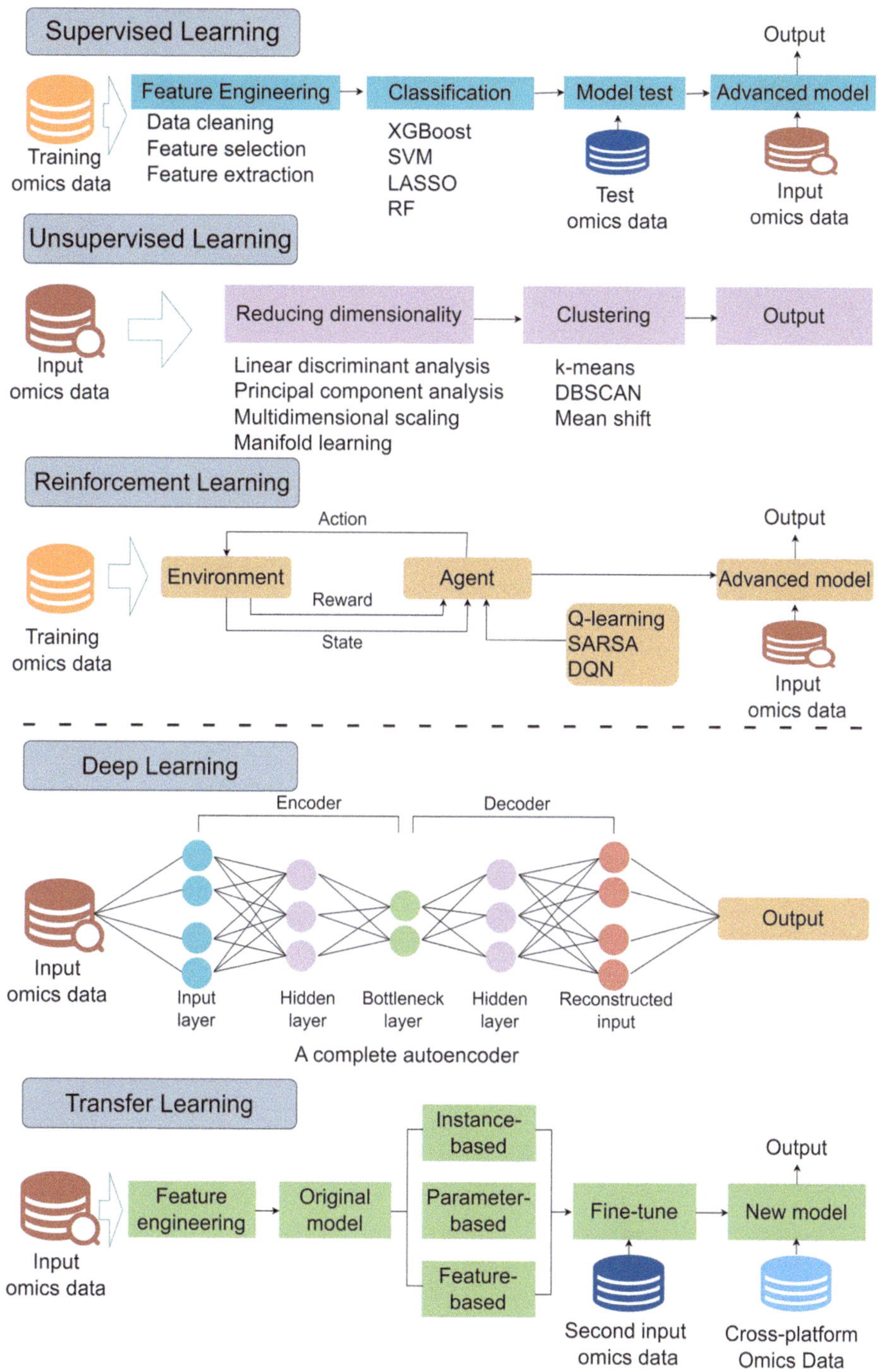

Fig. 3.2 Schematic of the ML pipeline in multi-omics studies

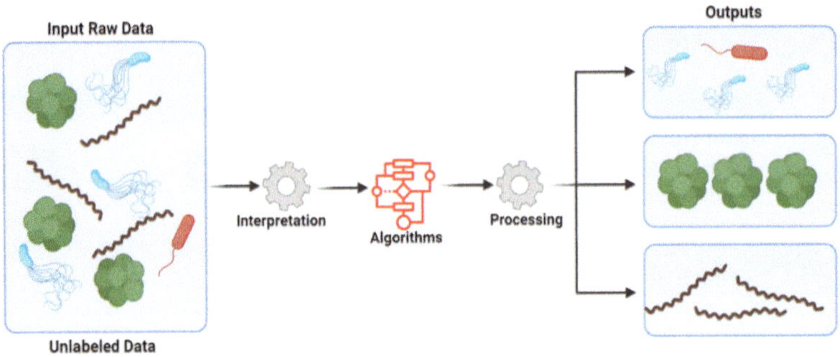

Fig. 3.3 Workflow for multi-omics integration and patient stratification using unsupervised learning and downstream predictive modeling

drug screening results, supervised algorithms can predict which new compounds are most likely to be successful or unsuccessful in clinical trials.

3.1.3 Use Cases across the Pipeline

AI has been effectively used at several phases of the medication development process, including:

- **Target Discovery:** New therapeutic targets linked to certain disease pathways can be found using AI models trained on genomic and pathway data [5].
- **Lead Optimization:** By forecasting activity, off-target effects, and ADME-Tox characteristics, machine learning methods optimize lead compounds for safety and efficacy.
- **Preclinical Testing:** It eliminates the need for expensive and time-consuming in vivo investigations by simulating pharmacokinetic (PK) and pharmacodynamic (PD) profiles.
- **Translational Research:** The discovery of biomarkers and patient stratification techniques is made possible by electronic health record (EHR) mining and multi-omics integration.

These applications highlight how AI can improve translational success by converting preclinical data into clinically useful insights.

3.1.4 A Shift Toward Precision and Personalization

The emergence of precision medicine, which tailor's treatments according to an individual's genetic, environmental, and lifestyle factors, has raised the demand for AI-driven technologies. Translational research is increasingly relying on the integration of multiple data kinds to develop complete models of disease. This integration is made easier by AI, which uncovers treatment options and molecular pathways that traditional approaches would miss [6].

Researchers at Google Health developed a DL algorithm that can directly predict cardiovascular risk from retinal images [7], demonstrating how AI may uncover hidden biomarkers across domains. Similarly, multi-modal AI models that combine imaging, clinical, and genomic data are being researched for cancer prognosis and treatment response prediction.

3.1.5 Ethical and Regulatory Considerations

The application of AI in preclinical and translational research presents significant obstacles despite its potential. Issues including algorithmic bias, repeatability, model interpretability, and data privacy need to be addressed to ensure that AI technologies are ethically and scientifically sound. Regulatory agencies such as the US Food and Drug Administration (FDA) and the European Medicines Agency (EMA) are actively developing frameworks for evaluating AI-based technologies in clinical practice and drug development.

Throughout the AI lifecycle, the FDA's "Good Machine Learning Practice" (GMLP) principles emphasize transparency, reliability, and human monitoring [8]. These guidelines will be crucial for ensuring the safe and reliable integration of AI systems into preclinical and translational procedures.

3.2 Predictive Toxicology and Pharmacokinetics

In drug development, efficient early-stage safety and pharmacokinetic (PK) evaluations are essential. High attrition throughout preclinical stages can be attributed to disappointing toxicity or subpar PK characteristics. This landscape is being transformed by AI-powered in silico tools that span predictive toxicology and PK/ADME modeling. These tools use machine learning (ML) and deep learning (DL) to effectively foresee adverse. Diverse chemical and biological databases serve as training sources, and advanced ML algorithms such as support vector machines, random forests, and deep neural networks are employed to analyze encoded molecular features. These predictions are further validated against in vitro or in vivo assays to assess outcomes like carcinogenicity, hepatotoxicity, and cardiotoxicity.

3.2.1 Predictive Toxicology

Background and Traditional Methods

Toxicological testing has traditionally used animal models and in vitro tests to detect risks such genotoxicity, cardiotoxicity, and hepatotoxicity. These techniques require a lot of resources, have ethical limitations, and frequently do not accurately forecast how people would react. The basis for AI-based methods has been established by the growth of publicly available toxicological databases, such as Tox21 and ToxCast.

ML and QSAR-Based Modeling

Toxicological endpoints are predicted using quantitative structure-activity relationship (QSAR) models using chemical descriptors generated from molecular structures. These include DL architecture as well as more conventional methods like random forest and support vector machines [9]. One significant development was DeepTox, a deep neural network that combined chemical descriptors and multitask learning to win the Tox21 Data Challenge. It proved that DL can automatically learn toxicophores and generalizable chemical characteristics by achieving AUCs that outperformed those of conventional ML techniques [10], as shown in Fig. 3.4, where hidden neurons successfully detect known toxicophores directly from chemical structures [10].

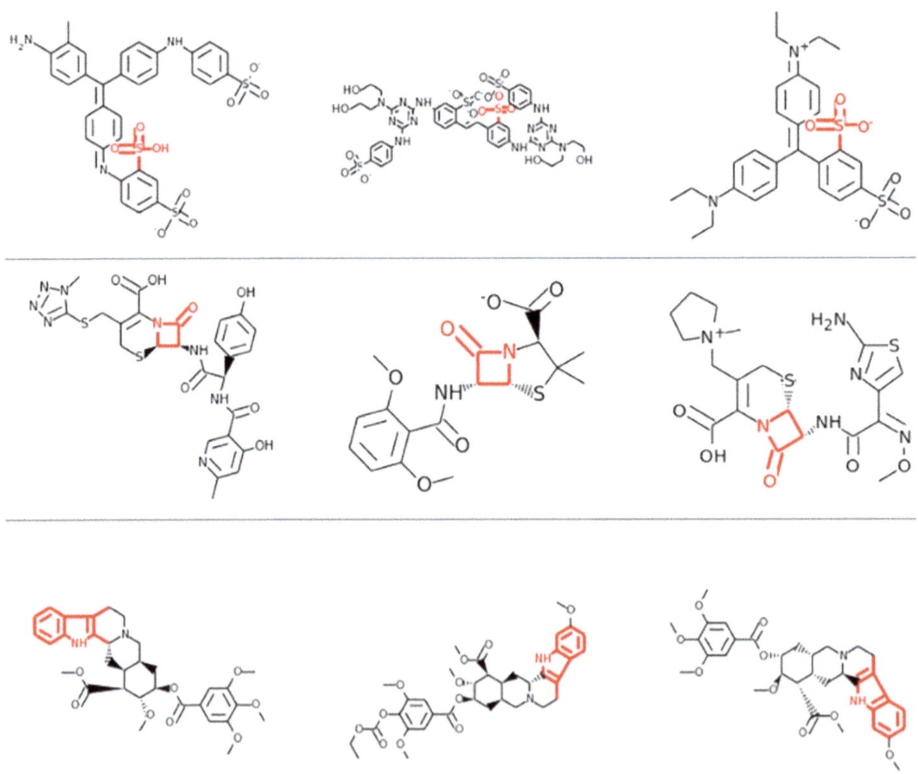

Fig. 3.4 Feature construction by deep learning. Neurons in the DeepTox model that have been learned to detect the presence of toxicophores substructures in chemical compounds

Case Studies and Ensemble Approaches

When it came to predicting nuclear receptors and stress-response toxicities, DeepTox performed better than conventional ML [10]. Graph convolutional networks (GCNs), fully connected neural networks, and Extreme Gradient Boosting (XGBoost) were all incorporated into a later ensemble model called Toxic Blend. On the Tox21 and ToxCast datasets, this hybrid technique produced state-of-the-art results [11].

Performance and Data Challenges

Dataset heterogeneity, interpretability, and dosage response quantification can be problems for even the most robust models. Although regulatory frameworks frequently demand dosage-related risk, most models concentrate on binary classification (toxic vs. nontoxic). Furthermore, comparing performance is made more difficult by inconsistent labeling between datasets.

Future Developments

- Enhanced descriptor engineering using autoencoders or molecular dynamics to capture complex chemical behavior [12].
- Ensemble pipelines integrating multitask learning to predict multiple toxicity endpoints simultaneously [10].
- Incorporation of human mechanistic data (e.g., transcriptomics, cellular imaging) via interpretable architectures to uncover toxicity pathways.

3.2.2 Predictive Pharmacokinetics and ADME-Tox

Importance in Drug Discovery

In more than 40% of clinical candidate failures, poor pharmacokinetics, absorption, distribution, metabolism, and excretion (ADME) are to blame. Conventional animal PK and in vitro research are expensive and time-consuming. AI provides quicker, less expensive, and frequently more accurate substitutes.

ML and PBPK Integration

To forecast PK parameters like clearance, AUC, half-life, and volume of distribution, machine learning models have been created. The most popular algorithms, according to a thorough study, are random forest and XGBoost, especially for clearance and AUC prediction [13]. At the same time, scalable, high-throughput predictions for sizable chemical libraries have been made using physiologically based pharmacokinetic (PBPK) modeling in conjunction with machine learning. It facilitates predictions across species and age groups as well as IVIVE (in vitro to in vivo extrapolation) [14].

Innovative Architectures

- **Chemi-Net**: A GCN model applied to physicochemical descriptors for PK property prediction, significantly outperforming Cubist regression models [15].
- **Transfer and Multitask Learning**: A neural approach predicting multiple PK parameters using pretrained bioactivity feature layers followed by multitask heads for parameters like bioavailability and half-life [16].

Editorial Perspectives

Recent editorials highlight AI's potential to disrupt ADME/Tox modeling by improving accuracy and reducing experimental demands. Frontiers in Drug Discovery emphasizes developing specific ADMET endpoint models, uncertainty quantification, interpretation, and integration into scoring systems [17].

Key Tools and Platforms

- **ADMET-AI**: A graph neural network-based platform predicting multiple ADMET endpoints from SMILES; ranked highly among benchmarks and capable of processing large compound batches.
- **Receptor.AI**: Employs multitask GCNs trained on datasets like ChEMBL and ToxCast to simultaneously predict toxicity and PK parameters, reducing candidate attrition in preclinical pipelines.

Table 3.1 shows the comparison of various prediction domains with strengths and challenges associated with them.

3.2.3 Integration of PK and Toxicity (ADMET-Tox)

PK profiles and toxicity are linked in drug development; a compound's buildup because of inadequate clearance might increase the likelihood of harm. To improve early-stage screening prioritizing, recent AI platforms employ multitask learning to predict both toxicity and PK parameters in unified models [14]. Candidate triage can be automated with an AI-based ADMET-Tox integration, balancing developability, safety, and efficacy.

Table 3.1 Comparison of various prediction domains

Domain	Techniques	Representative models	Strengths	Challenges
Toxicity prediction	QSAR, SVM, RF, DL, GCN, ensemble	DeepTox, ToxicBlend	High accuracy; multi-endpoint predictions	Predicting dose-response; data heterogeneity
PK/ADME modeling	RF, XGBoost, DL, PBPK+ML, multitask GCN	Chemi-net, ADMET-AI, receptor.AI	Scalable; covers multiple PK parameters	Model interpretability; uncertainty handling

3.2.4 Validation, Regulatory Context, and Challenges

Model Interpretability

Medicinal chemists and physicians are more likely to accept explainability strategies that aid in the interpretation of predictions, such as SHAP values and attention processes. Transparency in regulations still depends on interpretability.

Quality Datasets and Transfer Learning

Generalization requires:

- Transparent, high-quality datasets (e.g., Tox21, ChEMBL).
- Use of transfer learning to adapt pretrained models to proprietary chemical spaces.

Regulatory Considerations

Regulatory guidelines (FDA GMLP, EMA AI frameworks) emphasize:

- Input data quality.
- Transparent development processes.
- Validation against clinical samples.
- Human-in-the-loop oversight.

Transparency, auditability, and documented provenance throughout workflows are essential for compliance.

3.2.5 Outlook and Future Directions

- **Predictive Dose-Response Modeling:** Shift to classification models with quantal dose-response predictions.
- **Integration of Omics and High-Content Data:** Integrating transcriptomics, proteomics, and cellular phenotyping in identifying mechanistic information.
- **Model-Informed Precision Dosing (MIPD):** Integrating ML-PBPK predictions with individualized dosing regimens in the clinic [18].
- **Human-on-Chip and Bayesian Modeling:** Utilizing in vitro mini-organs and Bayesian models to enhance IVIVE modeling.
- **Federated Learning:** Co-training of a model by institutions with data privacy being preserved.

DL innovations, public data, graph neural models, and multitask architectures have all contributed to making preclinical AI reach full maturity in the field of toxicity and PK modeling. They enhance safety predictions, facilitate decision-making at the earliest possible time, and significantly speed up compound selection. Strong validation, interpretability, regulatory compliance, and smooth integration are key success drivers leading to truly predictive, mechanistically driven drug development.

3.3 Biomarker Identification

Biomarkers are biological indicators of disease status or treatment response that are integral to translational success. By facilitating high-dimensional data analysis from genomes, proteomics, imaging, and clinical records, artificial intelligence (AI), particularly machine learning (ML) and deep learning (DL), has significantly enhanced biomarker identification. Figure 3.5 shows a schematic diagram of digital biomarker research using deep-learning method [19]. Here, the preprocessed data can be used as digital biomarkers by extracting features through a deep neural network model, predicting the result, and evaluating it. Hidden layers can be composed by combining several types of layers according to functions and roles.

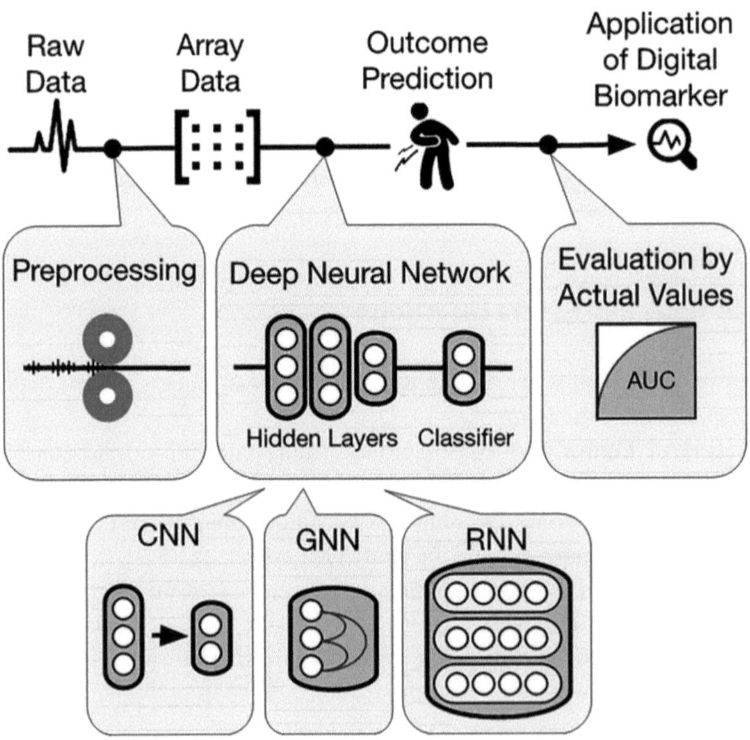

Fig. 3.5 Schematic diagram of digital biomarker research using deep learning method

3.3.1 Overview and Importance

Biomarkers are pivotal for:

- **Patient stratification**, enhancing treatment precision.
- **Predicting drug response**, reducing trial failure rates.
- **Monitoring disease progression**, enabling timely interventions.

Challenges include high-dimensional omics data, noise, and the need for interpretability. AI excels at uncovering nonlinear patterns beyond human identifiable.

3.3.2 Data Types and AI Approaches

- **Genomic and Transcriptomic Data**: RNA-seq and SNP arrays are examples of genomic and transcriptomic data. Common AI tools include clustering (k-means, hierarchical) for unsupervised patient subgroup discovery and random forests (RF), LASSO, and SVMs for supervised classification.
- **Proteomic and Metabolomic Data:** ML techniques such as logistic regression, RF, and DL autoencoders are used to process mass spectrometry data to reduce dimensionality and pick features.
- **Histopathological Imaging:** Ortega et al. (2022) employed convolutional neural networks (CNNs) on breast tissue scans to find prognostic patterns. CNNs uncover morphological traits that are linked to outcomes.
- **Clinical/EHR Data:** Longitudinal biomarkers are extracted from patient records using NLP and sequence models (LSTMs, transformers).

3.3.3 ML Techniques for Biomarker Discovery

Feature Selection and Dimensionality Reduction

- **Unsupervised techniques** for subgroup discovery and visualization include PCA, t-SNE, and UMAP.
- **Regularization techniques** for sparse feature selection include elastic net and LASSO.
- **Tree-based models**: ranking feature importance is provided by RF and gradient boosting machines (such as XGBoost).

Deep Learning Methods

- **Autoencoders and Variational Autoencoders (VAEs)** for embedding high-dimensional data into latent spaces that highlight biological variation.
- **Multi-modal DL** integrates omics, imaging, and clinical data. Merging features from autoencoders, CNNs, and MLPs enhance predictive performance.

3.3.4 Case Study: Oncology Biomarkers Evidence in Colorectal Cancer

The clinical evidence for each of the four modern personalized medicine biomarkers for colorectal cancer is examined in this case study, along with its assessment for inclusion in the NCCN Guidelines. The authors discovered that the published clinical evidence for these indicators is inconsistent and occasionally contradictory, suggesting that when developing guidelines, expert opinion, clinical judgment, and consensus frequently take precedence over clinical trial results.

There are advantages and disadvantages to depending on professional judgment. In contrast to more time-consuming guidelines based on formal systematic reviews, which may lag, it enables the immediate incorporation of developing data, as evidenced by the quick modification of B-raf recommendations following new discoveries [20]. According to a survey of 459 breast cancer surgeons, in the face of scientific uncertainty, expert opinion, followed by guidelines and consensus statements, strongly influences decision-making [21].

But bias is also a risk of this reliance. This danger is lessened by the NCCN's strict controls, which include conflict of interest disclosures, iterative panel assessment from a variety of specializations, and extensive institutional input [22, 23]. Notably, unlike the Oncotype DX Colon Cancer Assay, which NCCN has not accepted, the three suggested tests, K-ras and B-raf mutation analysis and MMR testing, are not proprietary.

There are still some possible subtle factors at play, such as the excitement around the discovery of the K-ras biomarker potentially skewing opinions about the evidence of the B-raf V600E mutation. Furthermore, because of things like research funding, patient advocacy, tumor-specific hazards, therapeutic efficacy, toxicity, and subspecialty biases, the threshold for biomarker suggestion may differ depending on the kind of cancer.

The difficulties in applying consistent evidence classifications to biomarkers are also highlighted by this study. K-ras, B-raf, and MMR tests were all rated as NCCN Category 2A despite varying data quality; however, the evidence supporting B-raf was significantly worse at inclusion. Due in part to challenges in selecting endpoints and differentiating between the functions of predictive and prognostic markers, biomarker studies—primarily retrospective subset analyses from case series, cohorts, and prospective randomized trials—fail to show discernible improvements in patient outcomes. For instance, B-raf V600E's unclear classification is hampered by the paucity of controlled research, which has led to changes in NCCN guidelines [24, 25].

Additionally, the release of preliminary findings at significant conferences such as the ASCO Annual Meeting sometimes occurs concurrently with the inclusion of NCCN guidelines, illustrating the interaction between expert consensus and evidence maturity. Although the focus was on biomarkers for individualized medicine, the same findings probably apply to other cutting-edge cancer treatments and technology that enter clinical usage before solid proof is available.

3.3.5 Deep Learning in Histopathology

In histopathology, deep learning has become a disruptive force by providing sophisticated techniques for tissue sample analysis and improving diagnostic precision. Tumor detection, classification, and prognostication are made easier using this method, which uses artificial intelligence (AI) to process intricate histology pictures [26]. As shown in Fig. 3.6, this process begins with whole-slide images (WSIs), which are divided into smaller image patches and analyzed using artificial neural networks to produce diagnostic and prognostic outputs.

In histopathology, convolutional neural networks (CNNs) are used to evaluate whole-slide images (WSIs) as part of the deep learning application. By learning to recognize and categorize different tissue patterns, these networks help pathologists more accurately identify cancers. CNNs, for example, have been used to distinguish between cancerous and non-cancerous cells with accuracy levels that are on par with or higher than those of human specialists. Additionally, deep learning models can predict patient outcomes and evaluate tumor heterogeneity, which helps guide treatment plans [26].

Despite these developments, there are still several obstacles to overcome before deep learning may be used in clinical settings. The training of strong models is hampered by the lack of annotated histopathology datasets. Furthermore, since comprehension of the reasoning behind model predictions is essential for clinical adoption, the interpretability of AI-driven judgments continues to be a challenge. Working together to create explainable AI frameworks and collect extensive datasets is necessary to address these problems [27].

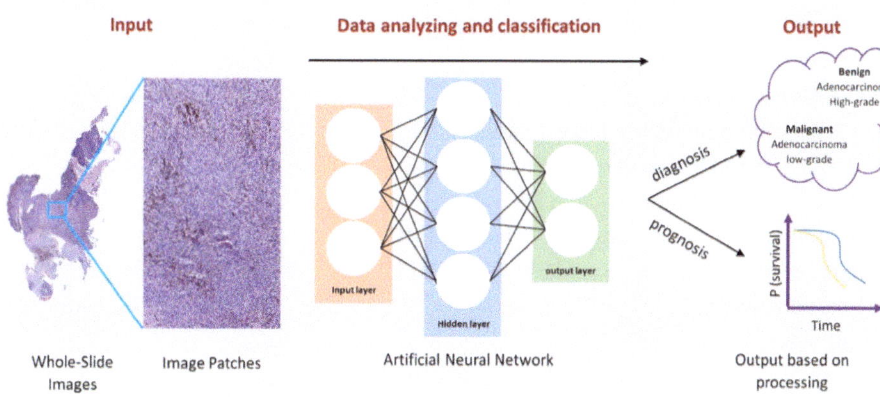

Fig. 3.6 An overview of the deep learning process in pathology. Firstly, the whole-slide images (WSIs) were obtained from the original specimen slides. Then, the ongoing artificial neural network (ANN) analysis process. Finally, the output of diagnosis or prognosis was based on the classification and selected features

3.3.6 Integrating Omics and Clinical Data

The combination of clinical and omics information is a significant step toward precision medicine that aims to provide tailored treatment by combining patient-specific clinical data with biological results. Integration enables the entire understanding of disease processes, which improves prognoses, diagnostics, and treatment.

The integration process entails bringing together clinical data, such as electronic health records (EHRs), with high-throughput omics data, such as transcriptomics, proteomics, metabolomics, and genomes. By identifying molecular signals for diseases, this pair improves prediction on what a disease will become and the effectiveness of the treatment. Analyzing such intricate information requires sophisticated computer methods, specifically machine learning and AI. From these techniques' capability of discovering hidden patterns and connections between the information, they help develop more accurate and tailored medical treatments.

While it holds promise, a variety of challenges are present in combining omics and clinical information. Combining is made difficult by data source diversity, data format diversity, as well as privacy and security concerns. Further, since clinical implementation necessitates the understanding of the reason behind model predictions, interpretability of AI models is a major challenge. To overcome these hurdles and make integrated studies reliable and transparent, there is a necessity to frame sound protocols, strong data governance systems, and explainable AI models.

3.3.7 Validation and Challenges

The validation strategies and challenges are as follows:

- **Validation Strategies:**
  - Cross-validation within large datasets.
  - Testing on independent cohorts.
  - Functional validation through lab assays.
  - Explainability techniques (e.g., SHAP, LIME).
  - Adherence to reporting standards like TRIPOD (for prognostic models), enhancing reproducibility.
- **Challenges:**
  - Risk of overfitting and lack of external validation.
  - Batch effects due to sample processing.
  - Ensuring model interpretability for clinical adoption.

3.4 Integration of Omics Data Using AI

Integrative multi-omics, which can include genomics, transcriptomics, proteomics, metabolomics, epigenomics, and increasingly histopathology and radiomics, has become a key element of precision medicine and translational science. The AI-enabled integrative approaches provide a systems-level view of disease by identifying complex and nonlinear relationships across many domains, while layers of omics essentially give useful but independent biological insights. In these integrations, artificial intelligence (especially deep learning and graph-based models) is most important. These forms of AI can establish and blend heterogeneous datasets across layers to align omics datasets even when some data are missing or have uneven data distribution (often called the "high dimensionality, sparsity, and heterogeneity" of the data) through models using multimodal transformers, deep canonical correlation analysis (DCCA), and variational autoencoders (VAEs) [28]. These models learn shared latent representations that expose shared regulatory networks and cross-omic biomarkers that are important for prognosis, identifying risk models and biomarker combinations that inform treatment responses, and subtyping diseases.

Moreover, AI-based integrative models have enabled rapid biomarker discovery in complex diseases such as cancer or neurodegeneration. They facilitate finding disease patterns across omics data and clinical features and can assist developing more standardized patient classification, increasing the efficiency of personalized treatment regimens [29]. As the volume and type of omics data increases, AI will continue to play a critical role in addressing the challenges associated with high dimensionality, sparsity, and heterogeneity and will continue closing the gap between bench and bedside.

3.4.1 The Challenge of Multi-Omics

Multi-omics data present significant computational challenges:

- **High dimensionality and heterogeneity**: Millions of features with distinct scales, distributions, and interdependence [30, 31].
- **Data missingness and sparsity**: Not all omics data are available for every sample, e.g., epigenomics may exist without proteomics.
- **Batch effects**: Variations from experimental or technical differences can obscure biological signals.

Emerging deep learning frameworks address these challenges using shared latent space learning, cross-modal attention mechanisms, and variational inference, which help reconcile data inconsistencies, extract joint representations, and uncover hidden regulatory interactions [29]. Overall, successful multi-omics integration demands flexible, robust AI techniques that preserve biological signal fidelity while navigating complex data structures.

3.4.2 Integration Strategies: Early, Intermediate, Late

Typical integration approaches include [32]:

- **Early fusion**: Raw data concatenation before modeling (e.g., deep feedforward networks).
- **Intermediate integration**: Each modality reduced separately and then fused (e.g., modality-specific autoencoders).
- **Late fusion**: Independent models per modality with results integrated (e.g., ensemble voting).

Advanced generative and graph-based models often use these hybrid approaches.

3.4.3 Statistical and Matrix Factorization Methods

- MOFA (multi-omics factor analysis) is a Bayesian factor analysis approach that captures both shared and modality-specific latent factors across omics datasets [33]. MOFA decomposes multiview data into latent factors and corresponding weights, enabling tasks such as variance decomposition, feature selection, clustering, and gene set enrichment analysis.
- MOFA+, MEFISTO, and single-cell MOFA2 are extensions of this framework, incorporating time-series or spatial data [33].
- Kernel/PCA-based concatenation methods offer simpler unsupervised alternatives but are less scalable for sparse or high-dimensional datasets.

These models provide interpretable representations of latent structure and variance sources, making them valuable for hypothesis generation and mechanistic insights.

3.4.4 Deep Learning Approaches

Recent advances in AI for multi-omics center around neural models:

Autoencoders and VAEs

- **Variational autoencoders (VAEs)** learn compressed multimodal embeddings, handle missing data, and correct batch effects [2, 31].
- **CustOmics**: A customizable autoencoder framework adaptively mixes modalities; shown effective in classification/survival tasks [34].
- **OmiEmbed**: A multitask deep embedding model achieving strong performance across classification, survival, and modality fusion [35].

Graph-Based Models

Graph neural networks (GNNs) encode biological networks:

- **DeepMOCCA** uses graph attention over multi-omics to enable pan-cancer survival predictions and biomarker discovery.
- **MoGCN** and other GCN-based models yield interpretable disease modules .

Hybrid Feedforward and CNN

- **MOLI**: Modality subnetworks merged via feedforward neural network, effective for drug response prediction.
- Other multi-omics DL approaches concatenate modality-specific embeddings for prognosis tasks [36].

3.4.5 Validation and Biological Interpretability

- **Latent Feature Validation**: Correlate with known biological annotations and pathway enrichment.
- **Joint Reconstruction Accuracy**: Test modality imputation.
- **Downstream Predictive Power**: Use learned embeddings in clinical outcome tasks.
- **Explainable AI (xAI)**: Techniques like SHAP and integrated gradients unveil feature contributions [37, 38].
- **Reproducibility standards** (e.g., rigorous external validation, clear preprocessing pipelines) are essential.

3.4.6 Future Directions

- **Foundation models and transformers**: Promising for cross-modal embedding's akin to large-scale language/image models.
- **Single-cell multi-omics**: Next frontier—modalities include scRNA-seq, ATAC-seq, CITE-seq; integration strategies continue evolving [36].
- **Federated learning**: Enables institution-spanning integration of sensitive patient datasets.
- **Integration beyond omics**: Linking omics with imaging, EHR, and wearable device data for richer phenotyping.

Descriptive models have given way to advanced embedding frameworks, autoencoders, GNNs, and generative architectures that handle data heterogeneity, uncover biomarkers, and represent complicated biology in AI-powered multi-omics integration. Although there are still issues with standardization, interpretability, and data sparsity, the development of foundation models and single-cell approaches puts this discipline in a position to make significant advances in translational medicine.

3.5 Challenges and Validation Strategies

While AI provides strong tools for translational and preclinical research, there are several obstacles that limit its practical use. Clinical trust and translational impact depend on model validity, interpretability, data integrity, and regulatory compliance.

3.5.1 Data Quality, Bias, and Generalizability

Data Limitations

- **Sparse and incomplete data** are common in multi-omics, toxicity, and PK datasets. Handling missingness through imputation or model architectures is critical but can introduce bias.
- **Batch effects** due to sample processing are major confounders. Methods like Combat and LIMMA are often used before AI modeling.
- **Label noise and measurement error** in experimental data undermine model performance. For instance, toxicity labels from different labs may use inconsistent thresholds.

Bias and Generalization

- Models trained on public datasets (e.g., Tox21) may not generalize to proprietary or clinical chemistries.
- Population bias in omics repositories (over-representation of European ancestry) limits model applicability to global populations.

Validation Strategies

- **External validation** on independent cohorts or chemotypes.
- **Cross-domain testing**, for example, training in rodents and testing on human cell data.
- **Stratified sampling** to ensure demographic and technical diversity.
- **Frequent recalibration** as new data emerges.

3.5.2 Interpretability and Explainability

AI models, especially deep neural networks, are often criticized as "black boxes." Interpretable models and explainable AI (xAI) methods are essential to understand decision logic for medicinal chemists, build clinician trust, and enable regulatory review. Key xAI techniques include:

- **Feature importance** (SHAP, LIME).
- **Attention mechanisms** in sequences/images.
- **Prototype-based methods**, e.g., testing with representative chemical structures or biological profiles.

Studies have shown that SHAP values can reliably mirror known toxicophores in DeepTox models.

3.5.3 Benchmarking and Reproducibility

A. **Reproducibility**: Frequently encountered obstacles include private datasets, undocumented preprocessing steps, and inaccessible code. Solutions:
   - Make use of open-source frameworks and code.
   - Exchange training metadata and model weights.
   - Make use of containerization (Singularity, Docker).

B. **Benchmarking:** A common test bed is provided via shared benchmarks, such as OpenPBTA for pediatric brain tumors and MoleculeNet for chemistry. They support model calibration and comparison across tasks and datasets.

3.5.4 Regulatory and Ethical Considerations

A. **Regulatory Landscape**
   - The **FDA's GMLP** outlines transparency, robustness, documentation, monitoring, and human review in AI/ML medical tools.
   - The **EMA** is developing AI-specific guidelines for medical devices and drug evaluation, emphasizing risk management and validation.

B. **Regulatory Compliance Demands**
   - **Input data traceability**.
   - **Clear documentation** of model design and training.
   - **Performance thresholds** based on clinical utility.
   - **Post-deployment monitoring** for drift and failures.

C. **Ethical Imperatives**
   - AI bias (ancestry, socioeconomic) must be actively tested and mitigated.
   - Patient privacy and data security are paramount in omics and EHR integration.
   - Consent must cover secondary data use, especially in federated learning and public-private partnerships.

Table 3.2 Validation metrics for performance evaluation

Criterion	Description
Statistical metrics	AUC, RMSE, precision/recall, calibration plots, confidence/uncertainty estimates
Biological relevance	Pathway enrichment, cell assay alignment, mechanistic consistency
Clinical/preclinical utility	Prospective cohorts; controlled studies testing AI-informed hypotheses
Robustness testing	Adversarial noise, input perturbations, out-of-distribution resilience

3.5.5 Deployment and Human-AI Collaboration

Successful translational AI involves:

- **Seamless integration** into workflows (e.g., chemists, toxicologists).
- **User-friendly software** with interactive explanation features.
- **Human-in-the-loop review**, combining AI triage with expert oversight.
- **Updatable models** to accommodate new biological insights.

3.5.6 Validation Metrics: Statistical and Biological

Validation should assess both statistical and biological performance given parameters in Table 3.2.

Models identifying biomarkers should undergo functional validation in vitro or in vivo, demonstrating biological utility of predictions.

3.5.7 Continuous Updating and Lifecycle Management

AI models are not static. Best practices include:

- **Version control** for code, data, and model checkpoints.
- **Retraining triggers** based on performance decay or new data.
- **Continuous monitoring** of input distributions and performance drift.
- **Governance frameworks**, involving multidisciplinary teams for risk oversight and review.

3.6 Summary

The convergence of translational, preclinical, and artificial intelligence research is changing the biomedical landscape. AI has become more than just a technical development; it is now a strategic imperative of contemporary drug research with applications from integrating multi-omics data to anticipating drug toxicity and pharmacokinetics to finding new biomarkers.

In this chapter, we looked at how AI might help early-stage R&D overcome persistent constraints. AI models like DeepTox and ensemble frameworks like ToxicBlend have outperformed conventional methods in predicting toxicology in terms of accuracy. AI-driven systems are making it possible to make faster and more accurate in silico predictions in pharmacokinetics and ADME-Tox modeling, which lessens the need for expensive animal models and increases the accuracy of early screening. Deep learning and multi-modal integration are providing biomarker discovery insights that are not possible to identify with conventional statistical methods alone. The integration of several omics' layers, genomic, transcriptomic, proteomic, and epigenomic, through AI frameworks like MOFA, DeepMOCCA, and autoencoders is arguably the most revolutionary, since it advances the potential of precision medicine.

Despite these accomplishments, the fundamental barriers to real-world use of AI models, including regulatory barriers, model interpretability, and quality of data, remain intact. Many AI models are developed in silico and are prepared under imagined scenarios, but do not generalize to clinical situations or real-world data. The challenges posed by overfitting models, batch effects, low reproducibility, and sparse data cannot be overstated. Further, ethical issues related to privacy, explainability, and bias must be actively managed, especially when AI tools are applied to inform decisions regarding human health. The future of AI in this area can be shaped in several important ways:

- **Moving Toward Biomedical Foundation Models:** Cross-task, cross-modal foundation models trained on a variety of biological data are becoming more popular in the biomedical AI industry, driven by large language models like GPT and foundation models like AlphaFold. These models can be effective, broadly applicable foundations for more specialized uses in drug response prediction, biomarker identification, and toxicology.
- **Federated and Privacy-Preserving AI's Ascent:** Federated learning alleviates limited data access and privacy concerns by allowing decentralized model training across institutions. In this model, raw patient data is never exchanged, which protects patient privacy and enhances model generalizability because models can be developed with the input of several institutions.
- **Spatial Multi-omics and Single-Cell:** Proteomics, spatial transcriptomics, single-cell RNA-seq, and ATAC-seq all offer novel computational hurdles as well as opportunities for artificial intelligence. It will take next-generation AI frameworks that surpass existing architectures to handle the tremendous dimensionality, noise, and temporal-spatial structure of these data kinds.
- **Regulatory Integration and Model Lifecycle Management:** AI models must be treated as evolving entities rather than static tools. A lifetime approach is necessary for this, including thorough training, ongoing observation, retraining, version control, and compliance auditing. Frameworks for assessing AI/ML-based tools are being actively developed by regulatory bodies like the FDA and EMA, with a focus on risk

management, explainability, model transparency, and Good Machine Learning Practice (GMLP).

- **Human-in-the-Loop Collaboration:** AI systems that work with domain experts rather than in place of them will be the most successful. Real-world settings are more likely to adopt tools that facilitate interactive exploration, offer explainable insights, and take expert feedback into account. Hybrid intelligence, which combines human judgment with mechanical precision, is the way of the future.

Artificial intelligence (AI) is disrupting both preclinical and translational research. The contemporary practice of biomedical science is evolving into a data-rich, maybe multi-modal and machine-augmented environment that is grounded solely in discovery, rather than only in hypothesis testing. The opportunities for preclinical and clinical research are multiplied, and while challenges remain, the writing is on the wall; AI will become progressively more instrumental in exploring the biological complexity of disease, facilitating the personalization of therapeutic interventions and developing our pathway from bench to bedside. It will require collaboration from all stakeholders in academic, business, and government settings to ensure the application of AI technology is ethical, explainable, and inclusive so that we can have a coherent and trustworthy transformation. Only then will it be possible for us to explore the promise of using AI in developing biomedical discoveries and improving public and planetary health.

References

1. DiMasi JA, Grabowski HG, Hansen RW. Innovation in the pharmaceutical industry: new estimates of R&D costs. J Health Econ. 2016;47:20–33. https://doi.org/10.1016/j.jhealeco.2016.01.012.
2. Lin M, Guo J, Gu Z, Tang W, Tao H, You S, Jia D, Sun Y, Jia P, et al. Machine learning and multi-omics integration: advancing cardiovascular translational research and clinical practice. J Transl Med. 2025;23:388. https://doi.org/10.1186/s12967-025-06425-2.
3. Esteva A, Robicquet A, Ramsundar B, et al. A guide to deep learning in healthcare. Nat Med. 2019;25:24–9. https://doi.org/10.1038/s41591-018-0316-z.
4. Chen R, Snyder M, Zhang K. The role of machine learning in precision medicine. Precis Clin Med. 2020;3(2):85–9. https://doi.org/10.1093/pcmedi/pbaa020.
5. Stokes JM, Yang K, Swanson K, et al. A deep learning approach to antibiotic discovery. Cell. 2020;180(4):688–702.e13. https://doi.org/10.1016/j.cell.2020.01.021.
6. Topol E. Deep medicine: how artificial intelligence can make healthcare human again. Basic Books; 2019.
7. Poplin R, Varadarajan AV, Blumer K, et al. Prediction of cardiovascular risk factors from retinal fundus photographs via deep learning. Nat Biomed Eng. 2018;2(3):158–64. https://doi.org/10.1038/s41551-018-0195-0.
8. FDA. Good machine learning practice for medical device development: guiding principles. U.S. Food and Drug Administration; 2021. https://www.fda.gov/medical-devices/software-medical-device-samd/good-machine-learning-practice-medical-device-development-guiding-principles

9. Wikipedia contributors. Quantitative structure–activity relationship. Wikipedia. https://en.wikipedia.org/wiki/Quantitative_structure%E2%80%93activity_relationship. Accessed 21 June 2025.
10. Mayr A, Klambauer G, Unterthiner T, Hochreiter S. DeepTox: toxicity prediction using deep learning. Front Environ Sci. 2016;3:80. https://doi.org/10.3389/fenvs.2015.00080.
11. Zaslavskiy M, Jégou S, Tramel EW, Wainrib G. ToxicBlend: virtual screening of toxic compounds with ensemble predictors. arXiv:1806.04449 [stat.ML]; 2018 Jun 12.
12. Wikipedia. ARKA descriptors in QSAR. In: *Wikipedia, The Free Encyclopedia*. https://en.wikipedia.org/wiki/ARKA_descriptors_in_QSAR. Accessed 21 June 2025.
13. Ahmadi M, Alizadeh B, Ayyoubzadeh SM, et al. Predicting pharmacokinetics of drugs using artificial intelligence tools: a systematic review. Eur J Drug Metab Pharmacokinet. 2024;49:249–62. https://doi.org/10.1007/s13318-024-00883-7.
14. Lin Z, Chou WC. Machine learning and artificial intelligence in toxicological sciences. Toxicol Sci. 2022;189(1):7–19. https://doi.org/10.1093/toxsci/kfac075.
15. Liu K, Sun X, Jia L, Ma J, Xing H, Wu J, Gao H, Sun Y, Boulnois F, Fan J. Chemi-net: a graph convolutional network for accurate drug property prediction arXiv:1803.06236 [cs.LG]; 2018 Mar 16. https://doi.org/10.48550/arXiv.1803.06236.
16. Ye Z, Yang Y, Li X, Cao D, Ouyang D. An integrated transfer learning and multitask learning approach for pharmacokinetic parameter prediction. arXiv:1812.09073 [cs.LG, stat.ML]; 2018 Dec 21.
17. Brogi S, Schyman P, Siramshetty VB. Editorial: pharmacokinetics modeling in the artificial intelligence era. Front Drug Discov. 2025;5:1636070. https://doi.org/10.3389/fddsv.2025.1636070.
18. Wikipedia. Model-Informed Precision Dosing. In: *Wikipedia, The Free Encyclopedia*. https://en.wikipedia.org/wiki/ModelInformed_Precision_Dosing. Accessed 22 June 2025.
19. Jeong H, Jeong YW, Park Y, Kim K, Park J, Kang DR. Applications of deep learning methods in digital biomarker research using noninvasive sensing data. Digit Health. 2022;8:20552076221136642. https://doi.org/10.1177/20552076221136642.
20. Somerfield MR, Einhaus K, Hagerty KL, et al. American Society of Clinical Oncology clinical practice guidelines: opportunities and challenges. J Clin Oncol. 2008;26:4022–6.
21. Schroen AT, Brenin DR. Breast cancer treatment beliefs and influences among surgeons in areas of scientific uncertainty. Am J Surg. 2010;199:491–9.
22. National Comprehensive Cancer Network. About the NCCN Clinical Practice Guidelines in Oncology. http://www.nccn.org/professionals/physician_gls/about.asp. Accessed 1 Dec 2010.
23. National Comprehensive Cancer Network. NCCN disclosure policies and potential conflicts of interest. http://www.nccn.org/about/disclosure.asp. Accessed 1 Dec 2010.
24. Engstrom PF, Arnoletti JP, Benson AB III, et al. NCCN Clinical Practice Guidelines in Oncology: Colon Cancer Version 2, 2010. http://www.nccn.org/professionals/physician_gls/PDF/colon.pdf. Accessed 1 Dec 2010.
25. Van Cutsem E, Lièvre A, Folprecht G, Nowacki M, et al. Cetuximab plus FOLFIRI in the treatment of metastatic colorectal cancer (mCRC): the influence of KRAS and BRAF biomarkers on outcome: updated data from the CRYSTAL trial. Presented at the 2010 ASCO gastrointestinal cancers symposium; 22–24 Jan 2010; Orlando, FL.
26. Ahmed AA, Abouzid M, Kaczmarek E. Deep learning approaches in histopathology. Cancers (Basel). 2022;14(21):5264. https://doi.org/10.3390/cancers14215264.
27. Li X, Zhang Y, Zhang S, et al. Deep learning of histopathology images at the single cell level. Front Artif Intell. 2021;4:754641. https://doi.org/10.3389/frai.2021.754641.
28. Zitnik M, Leskovec J. Predicting multicellular function through multi-layer tissue networks. Bioinformatics. 2017;33(14):i190–8. https://doi.org/10.1093/bioinformatics/btx252.

29. Chaudhary K, Poirion OB, Lu L, Garmire LX. Deep learning-based multi-omics integration robustly predicts survival in liver cancer. Clin Cancer Res. 2018;24(6):1248–59. https://doi.org/10.1158/1078-0432.CCR-17-0853.
30. Yates J, Van Allen EM. New horizons at the interface of artificial intelligence and translational cancer research. Cancer Cell. 2025;43(4):708–27. https://doi.org/10.1016/j.ccell.2025.03.002.
31. Baião AR, Cai Z, Poulos RC, Robinson PJ, Reddel RR, Zhong Q, Vinga S, Gonçalves E. A technical review of multi-omics data integration methods: from classical statistical to deep generative approaches. arXiv:2501.17729 [q-bio.QM]; 2025 Jan 29. https://doi.org/10.48550/arXiv.2501.17729
32. Wikipedia. Single-cell multi-omics integration. In: *Wikipedia, The Free Encyclopedia*. Published early June 2025. https://en.wikipedia.org/wiki/Single-cell_multi-omics_integration. Accessed 23 Jun 2025.
33. Argelaguet R, Velten B, Arnol D, et al. Multi-omics factor analysis—a framework for unsupervised integration of multi-omics data sets. Mol Syst Biol. 2018;14(6):e8124. https://doi.org/10.15252/msb.20178124.
34. Benkirane H, Pradat Y, Michiels S, Cournède PH. CustOmics: a versatile deep-learning based strategy for multi-omics integration. arXiv:2209.05485 [q-bio.GN, cs.LG]; 2022 Sep 12. https://doi.org/10.48550/arXiv.2209.05485
35. Zhang X, Xing Y, Sun K, Guo Y. OmiEmbed: a unified multi-task deep learning framework for multi-omics data. arXiv:2102.02669 [q-bio.GN]; 2021 Feb 3 (v1), revised 2021 May 18 (v2). https://doi.org/10.48550/arXiv.2102.02669
36. Ballard JL, Wang Z, Li W, Shen L, Long Q. Deep learning-based approaches for multi-omics data integration and analysis. BioData Min. 2024;17(1):38. https://doi.org/10.1186/s13040-024-00391-z.
37. Tang M. Multi-omics integration strategy and deep diving into MOFA2. Diving into Genetics and Genomics [blog] June 2025. https://divingintogeneticsandgenomics.com/post/multiomics-mofa2/. Accessed 23 Jun 2025.
38. Argelaguet R, Arnol D, Bredikhin D, et al. MOFA+: a statistical framework for comprehensive integration of multi-modal single-cell data. Genome Biol. 2020;21(1):111. https://doi.org/10.1186/s13059-020-02015-1.

Machine Learning in Clinical Trial Design and Optimization

4

Clinical trials remain the gold standard for evaluating new therapies, but they are notoriously slow, expensive, and often fail due to poor design and patient mismatch. Trials are "complex, labor-intensive, [and] expensive," and failure is frequently blamed on "poor patient cohort selection and recruiting mechanisms" [1]. In response, researchers are applying AI and machine learning (ML) to reshape trial design. As Zhang et al. note, AI has "unparalleled potential to unlock useful information from real-world data to innovate trial design." In practical terms, this means using ML to analyze large health datasets and simulate alternatives, for example, tools like Trial Pathfinder apply electronic health records to identify overly strict inclusion rules. In one case, relaxing certain eligibility criteria (e.g., lab value cutoffs) doubled the pool of eligible patients in a lung cancer trial while maintaining outcomes [1]. More generally, adaptive and data-driven methods are beginning to transform every stage of trials.

4.1 Patient Stratification and Recruitment

4.1.1 ML-Based Patient Stratification to Improve Statistical Power

A critical challenge in trials is patient heterogeneity. Different individuals may respond very differently to the same treatment, diluting observable effects. Machine learning can identify homogeneous subgroups or predictive biomarkers to enrich trials with patients most likely to benefit. For example, in Alzheimer's disease, Birkenbihl et al. used a deep-learning model to cluster patients by their longitudinal symptom trajectories. The model split early-stage patients into "fast" and "slow" progressors. Trials enriched with the faster-declining subgroup achieved the same statistical power with far fewer patients [2].

K. Shaikh et al., *Artificial Intelligence in Drug Discovery and Development*,
Synthesis Lectures on Engineering, Science, and Technology,
https://doi.org/10.1007/978-3-032-10277-5_4

In fact, the researchers estimated that targeting faster progressors could reduce sample size by >13% and lower costs substantially [2]. Each patient's time course of cognitive scores is used to predict subgroup membership, and enrolling the high-risk "fast" group yields a smaller, more efficient cohort [2].

Other examples abound. In critical care, Phillips et al. analyzed over 50,000 ICU patients with acute respiratory distress syndrome (ARDS) and used a gradient-boosting ML model to predict which patients would have prolonged ICU courses ("long-stay" subgroup) versus rapid recovery or death. By enrolling only those likely to stay and be assessable, trial statistical power increases. In simulation, their algorithm identified the long-stay subgroup with good accuracy (AUC $\approx$ 0.77) and, as they describe, "can identify patients with sufficiently long ARDS episodes to allow time for patients to respond to therapy, increasing statistical power" [3]. They also note that ML-based early-alert systems could actively flag eligible patients in real time, potentially improving recruitment rates. Similarly, in cardiovascular trials, Oikonomou et al. developed a "phenomapping" approach: at pre-planned interim analyses, an ML model learned patient phenotypes predictive of treatment benefit. By then conditionalizing enrollment probability on predicted benefit, they projected ~15–18% smaller trials without changing the observed treatment effect [4]. In short, ML-driven stratification (sometimes called predictive enrichment) leverages complex patient data (clinical features, genomics, imaging, etc.) to focus on those most likely to have measurable benefit [3, 4].

These AI-based stratification methods effectively "make better use of resources," as adaptive design advocates describe—often yielding more efficient and ethical trials [5]. In oncology, for instance, radiomics and computational pathology are being used to select patients with tumor characteristics. Azenkot et al. specifically note that "AI-powered diagnostic tools, including radiomics, computational pathology, and spatial omics, can improve trial patient selection and response assessments" [6]. Likewise, dozens of recent studies have shown that multimodal AI markers can serve as inclusion criteria to shrink required sample sizes while maintaining power. In essence, ML creates virtual biomarkers (from images, labs, or genetic data) that allow trials to enroll a more homogeneous group. As Zhang et al. explains, using rich real-world data to refine eligibility can even uncover patients who should qualify: their analysis with Trial Pathfinder found that 70% of patients who benefited were excluded under traditional criteria [1].

Beyond enrichment, AI also streamlines recruitment. Automated matching systems parse electronic health records (EHRs) and trial protocols to find candidate participants. Modern matching tools use natural language processing and machine learning to interpret both clinical notes and trial eligibility rules. For example, Hassanzadeh et al. proposed an algorithm that automatically scores how well each patient matches a given trial. In practice, such systems have demonstrated high accuracy in oncology settings: multiple studies report that ML-driven matching can reliably screen thousands of cancer patients for eligible trials [1]. By pre-screening or flagging patients who meet complex criteria, AI can greatly speed up accrual. Indeed, patient accrual is the leading cause of trial delays and failures, and even modest gains in matching efficiency can have large impact.

AI further supports patient-centric recruitment and monitoring. Integrating data from wearables, mobile apps, or social media, ML can broaden outreach and engage underrepresented groups. For instance, Zhang et al. note that patient-centric tools (apps, digital campaigns) improve trial access and diversity [1], and AI can help target those tools more intelligently. Data from digital health technologies—such as smartphone sensors or electronic diaries—"may enable a more comprehensive understanding of patient populations to support clinical trials from enrollment to assessment" [6]. In practice, ML models can analyze this real-world data to identify subpopulations who could benefit or to continuously monitor patients during the trial. AI-driven predictive analytics can even forecast dropout risk or adverse events, allowing investigators to intervene or adjust follow-up. As Azenkot et al. summarize by integrating AI/ML, trials become "more adaptive, data-driven, and inclusive." In short, machine learning is enabling smarter recruitment—matching the right patients to the right trials more quickly and ensuring enrolled cohorts are representative and engaged [1, 6].

Machine learning (ML) is transforming how clinical trials are planned and conducted by uncovering complex patterns in patient data. A major benefit is **patient stratification**: ML can divide a traditionally heterogeneous trial population into more homogeneous subgroups. This improves statistical power and can dramatically reduce the number of patients needed. For example, Schwager et al. showed that by training an ML model on an enormous ICU dataset (51,555 ARDS patients), they could predict which patients would have prolonged acute respiratory distress syndrome (ARDS) courses. By focusing enrollment on those "long-stay" patients, the study boosted trial power through cohort homogeneity [3]. The authors demonstrated feasibility of *prospective* ML-based stratification in ARDS, identifying long-ARDS patients so that therapies have time to take effect, thereby reducing the required sample size and *increasing* statistical power. They even proposed real-time alerts to recruit such patients as they present, thereby speeding enrollment. In short, ML-directed stratification turns a "one-size-fits-all" design into a targeted trial: subpopulations are defined by their predicted disease trajectories or biomarker profiles, and each is treated as its own mini-trial cohort. This approach has been shown to markedly improve efficiency in difficult settings (ICU, oncology, etc.), where heterogeneity has historically doomed many studies [3, 6].

4.1.2 High-Dimensional Data and Predictive Features for Trial Enrichment

In practice, ML-driven stratification uses high-dimensional data (genomics, imaging, vital signs, lab values, electronic health records) to detect hidden patient phenotypes. For instance, modern AI methods like ensemble models or deep learning can identify complex combinations of features that predict response or resistance to a therapy. These predictive features are then used to "enrich" the trial population. A recent review highlights that ML simulations of patient outcomes can *enhance stratification strategies* and thus statistical power. Likewise, advanced diagnostic tools—such as radiomics and spatial "omics"—are being combined with ML to pre-screen patients whose tumors or disease characteristics best match the investigational treatment [6]. In oncology, for example, AI-based image analysis can flag patients whose tumor genetics make them likely responders, thereby defining inclusion criteria more precisely. By front-loading this stratification step, trials can enroll only those individuals most likely to benefit, sidestepping the usual dilution of effects caused by nonresponders. Such enrichment strategies—often referred to as *precision* or *adaptive enrichment* designs—have been simulated in large cardiovascular trials and shown to cut required enrollment by roughly 15–18% while preserving the observed treatment effect [4]. In that study, the algorithm created a multidimensional "phenomap" of participants at interim analyses and then biased future enrollment toward candidates with the strongest predicted benefit, effectively making each new patient "more valuable" to the trial outcome [4, 6].

4.1.3 AI for Efficient Patient Recruitment and Matching

Machine learning also greatly streamlines patient recruitment, another major bottleneck. Instead of relying on manual chart review or traditional advertising, AI tools can sift through electronic health records (EHR), genomic databases, and other clinical data to identify eligible patients. For example, commercial platforms like IBM Watson for Clinical Trial Matching and Mendel.ai use natural language processing (NLP) and ML to parse unstructured clinical notes and match patients to trial protocols [7]. In practice, these systems can automatically flag potential candidates by scanning for eligibility criteria in real time. A recent scoping review of 51 AI-recruitment studies found overwhelmingly positive outcomes: trials using AI saw *increased efficiency, cost savings, faster recruitment, and improved accuracy* in finding patients. Patients also reported higher satisfaction when enrollment processes were guided by intelligent matching systems, which can provide clearer rationale and easier pre-screening than traditional methods [7].

Behind these successes is the ability of AI to recognize subtle patterns. For example, ML models can combine dozens of factors (age, labs, vital trends, genetics, etc.) to predict who will meet inclusion criteria before clinicians realize it. One trial even simulated hourly ICU screenings with an ML algorithm to flag septic shock onset, marking patients eligible the moment they qualify for a study. In general, by leveraging knowledge discovery and NLP on EHR and literature, AI enables "efficient participant matching" well ahead of enrollment. Indeed, AI can automatically extract key eligibility information from the vast free text in trial registries and patient records, essentially "pre-computing" trial lists for each patient and vice versa [7]. Once flagged, patients can be approached more quickly, and sites spend less time on fruitless screening. In effect, ML reallocates recruitment effort to the most promising leads, cutting down overhead and delays.

4.1.4 AI for Patient Monitoring, Retention, and Trial Optimization

Beyond recruitment, ML holds promise for retention and monitoring, although this is still emerging. Intelligent systems can use wearable and sensor data to detect signs of patient dropout or non-adherence, triggering personalized follow-ups. AI-driven chatbots and apps are being tested to engage participants with reminders and education, which early evidence suggests may improve compliance. While rigorous studies of AI for retention are fewer than for recruitment, the underlying capability is clear: continuous data capture (via smartphones or IoT devices) fed into predictive models can spot patients at risk of leaving a study and allow early intervention. Such integrated digital tools may be an important extension of ML-driven trial optimization, ensuring that the right patients stay in the trial long enough to reach endpoints.

Overall, ML is helping to humanize and tailor clinical trial design. By analyzing complex medical histories and biomarkers, it can group patients into biologically meaningful segments, ensuring each cohort is internally consistent. It also automates the matching of patients to trials, respecting individual characteristics. Through these functions, AI and ML attack two of the hardest parts of trial setup: identifying the right patients and doing so quickly and cheaply. As one recent review notes, the focus of AI in trials has rightly been on Phase II/III studies, where stratification and sample-size issues are most acute [6]. In these later-phase trials, better patient selection and recruitment can directly translate into better power and shorter timelines, benefiting both science and patient welfare.

4.2 Adaptive Trail Design Using AI

4.2.1 Introduction to Adaptive Trail Designs and the Role of AI

Adaptive clinical trial designs allow pre-planned, data-driven modifications during the trial (such as changing sample size, arm allocation, or even the patient population) to improve efficiency and ethics. By using accumulating data to guide mid-course corrections, adaptive trials can conserve resources and reduce patient exposure compared to fixed designs. Recent reviews emphasize that adaptive designs can be more efficient, informative and ethical, often requiring fewer participants for the same power [4, 5]. The FDA has explicitly recognized this: guidance suggests that after an interim look, "a decision will be made based on prespecified criteria whether to continue enrollment in the overall population or to restrict future enrollment to the targeted subpopulation." In practice, however, identifying optimal adaptations (and validating them) is complex. This is where AI/ML can play a transformative role.

One clear application is predictive enrichment within an adaptive framework. As noted above, ML models can learn which patients are most likely to benefit and then adapt to enrollment accordingly. Oikonomou et al. implemented this via "phenomapping" in cardiovascular trials: at each interim analysis, their ML model identified phenotypic signatures of treatment benefit; then in simulations, they increased the probability of enrolling patients with high predicted benefit. This adaptive predictive enrichment reduced the projected final sample sizes by ~15–18% while preserving the original treatment effect (hazard ratios remained virtually unchanged). In other words, by focusing on the most responsive patients' mid-trial, statistical power was maintained even with far fewer subjects [4]. This approach echoes FDA-advised enrichment strategies and highlights how AI can operate them.

4.2.2 AI for Trial Simulation, Design Optimization, and Adaptive Randomization

AI can also inform trial simulation and design upfront. Computational tools like Trial Pathfinder (above) effectively perform hundreds of virtual trials under different scenarios, revealing which design choices matter. For example, by simulating completed lung cancer trials, Trial Pathfinder showed that relaxing certain lab-value inclusion rules could double eligible patients without diluting the effect [1]. This kind of data-driven simulation can be used before a trial starts to set optimal inclusion/exclusion criteria, allocate sample size, or identify key covariates to balance. Similarly, ML can be embedded in response-adaptive randomization or dose-finding. In principle, techniques like reinforcement learning (RL) could treat each patient's assignment as a "decision" to be optimized: an RL agent could learn over time which treatment is working better and skew future randomization accordingly. While still mostly theoretical, a recent primer notes that RL's ability to "continuously learn from data can significantly improve clinical trial outcomes," by optimizing sequential decisions [8]. For example, an RL framework might adaptively select doses or arm allocations to maximize overall patient benefit as the trial progresses. Though adaptive randomization and bandit algorithms have been proposed for years, combining them with modern ML and large datasets may finally make them viable in practice.

4.2.3 Virtual Control Arms and Digital Twin Patients

Another frontier is virtual control arms and digital twins. Building on enrichment and randomization, some AI platforms create synthetic comparator data to boost power. For instance, a company called Unlearn is developing TwinRCTs, which uses historical data and ML-generated "digital twin" patients for the control arm [1]. Each enrolled patient has a simulated counterpart under standard treatment, so fewer real patients need to be randomized to placebo. In theory this can greatly shorten enrollment and increase patient appeal (fewer receive placebo) while still preserving statistical rigor. Zhang et al. discuss this approach and note that regulators (e.g., the European Medicines Agency) have even suggested digital twins could be used in Phase II/III analyses without introducing bias.

Such innovations illustrate how AI can make trial execution fundamentally more flexible and efficient.

4.2.4 Challenges, Ethics, and Regulatory Considerations in AI-Driven Adaptive Trials

Of course, integrating AI into adaptive trials carries challenges. All adaptations must preserve trial validity and control false positives. It is therefore critical to validate ML models thoroughly. Encouragingly, in the examples above the ML-driven adaptations did not skew the results: Oikonomou et al. report that their enriched trial preserved the original hazard ratio ($p < 0.01$ in simulations) [4]. At the same time, AI-driven designs raise questions of transparency and fairness. As one review cautions, any ML tool in trials must be "explainable, ethical, repeatable, and scalable." More recently, Azenkot et al. emphasize the need to "mitigate bias and uphold ethical use" of AI in clinical research [6]. Regulatory bodies are actively considering this as well. The FDA and other agencies are developing guidance on AI/ML in drug development, and FDA's draft guidance on digital twins highlights the requirement that any synthetic arm not introduce systematic bias [1]. In practice, successful use of AI will require high-quality data (standardized EHRs, images, etc.), careful statistical planning, and ongoing monitoring.

In summary, machine learning is enabling a new generation of adaptive trial designs that are more flexible, efficient, and patient-centered. By stratifying patients, personalizing enrollment, simulating outcomes, and generating synthetic controls, AI has the potential to dramatically improve trial success rates and speed. While many of these ideas are still emerging, early studies demonstrate clear gains: ML-based enrichment can reduce trial size by on the order of 15–20% [4, 5], and AI-enabled recruitment tools have already accelerated patient matching in practice. As technology and data access continue to grow, these methods will likely become integral to trial design. Researchers and regulators alike agree that the future of clinical trials will be more adaptive and data-driven—and machine learning will be at the heart of this transformation.

4.2.5 ML-Based Adaptive Designs: From Predictive Enrichment to Reinforcement Learning and beyond

Unlike fixed "one-size-fits-all" trials, adaptive trial designs allow pre-planned modifications based on accumulating data. Examples include changing the randomization ratio, dropping inferior treatment arms, or adjusting sample size and endpoints. Incorporating AI into adaptive designs takes this flexibility even further. ML models can continuously learn from interim results and recommend design changes in real time. For instance, AI-driven adaptive designs can trigger unscheduled analyses or switch target populations the moment a safety or efficacy trend emerges [6]. This makes trials far more responsive: rather than passively waiting until the end, the study "listens" to the data and adapts on-the-fly.

Another study in cardiovascular trials used XGBoost models at interim analyses to estimate each new patient's likely benefit, then *conditioned the enrollment probability on that estimate*. They found that, by enrolling more "promising" patients as identified by the ML model, the final required sample size would have been roughly 15–18% smaller compared to a standard design while maintaining the original treatment effect size. In other words, AI allowed an ongoing trial to focus resources on the candidates most likely to improve efficacy estimates, making the trial more efficient without biasing the results.

More generally, ML enables real-time modifications that go beyond classic adaptive rules. In traditional adaptive designs, one might update the sample size or stop the trial early for futility. With AI, one can also adapt to the *target population* or *enrollment pace* dynamically. For instance, Bayesian or reinforcement-learning algorithms can adjust randomization probabilities in response to accumulating outcomes, a sort of "multi-armed bandit" approach where better-performing arms get more patients. In reinforcement learning (RL) terms, each patient assignment is an "action," and the algorithm learns a policy to maximize some objective (e.g., patient benefit). Early work showed that Q-learning and related RL techniques can derive optimal sequential treatment strategies directly from clinical trial data without needing an explicit mathematical model [9]. This means an RL-based trial design could sequentially adapt multi-stage regimens (multiple lines of therapy) by learning from observed outcomes, a potentially powerful method in oncology or chronic disease trials. Although still mostly in the research stage, such RL frameworks promise a way to personalize trial conduct itself: each new patient's assignment can be chosen not just by chance or simple rules, but by a learned algorithm that anticipates long-term benefits.

Machine learning can also simulate and optimize protocols before or during a trial. "Digital twin" technology is an emerging example: by generating a synthetic copy of each patient's likely disease course, sponsors can run *virtual clinical trials* to test design options. These in silico trials let researchers tweak inclusion criteria, dosing schedules, or analysis plans and see how outcomes might change—effectively using ML to stress-test the protocol. In one high-profile case, digital-twin models retrospectively applied to a failed Alzheimer's trial produced individual outcome forecasts that closely matched reality. The analysis showed that, had those predictions been used prospectively as covariate adjustments, the trial could have reduced its sample size by about 10% without altering the conclusions. While formal guidance on digital twins is still evolving, regulators are beginning to accept them to sharpen efficacy estimates and reduce variability [10].

Finally, AI can support decentralized and complex designs that would be infeasible otherwise. For example, in basket trials (testing one drug in multiple subpopulations) or platform trials (testing multiple drugs in one disease), ML tools can help decide when to add or drop arms. If interim data shows a new mutation-defined subgroup responding, an AI system could signal to open a new cohort; conversely, poor performance could close an arm early. Wearable sensors and mobile apps provide streams of patient data (heart rate, activity, etc.) that AI can fuse with clinical endpoints in real time. This data fusion can trigger adaptations—for instance, automatically switching a trial endpoint if sensor data indicate an emerging surrogate marker. The overall effect is a trial that "learns" from itself. In the words of a recent review, AI integration will make trials more adaptive, data-driven, and inclusive, enabling changes on-the-fly to improve patient outcomes and trial efficiency [6].

4.3 Real-Time Data Analysis and Monitoring

4.3.1 Real-Time Data Collection in Modern Clinical Trials

Continuous real-time data gathering and analysis are becoming more essential to trial design and supervision in modern clinical research. While manual data aggregation and sporadic site visits were common in traditional clinical trials, advancements in digital health technology have made it possible to continuously monitor participant data streams in real time. For instance, physiological signals (heart rate, activity, temperature, etc.) can be instantly recorded by wearable sensors and mobile health devices and sent to centralized databases. This change eliminates the need for recurring reporting and enables researchers and doctors to monitor patient condition "on the fly." According to Shajari et al., wearables with AI capabilities offer a "non-invasive and comfortable approach of monitoring patient health" by continuously measuring a range of biomarkers. By enabling early detection of negative trends (like an arrhythmia seen by a smart watch) and monitoring patient adherence to protocols (like medication regimens) through connected applications or ingestion sensors, such real-time collecting enhances safety and compliance [11, 12].

4.3.2 AI-Driven Data Analysis and Risk-Based Monitoring

Utilizing this real-time data requires the use of AI and machine learning. Compared to manual inspection, automated algorithms can continuously examine incoming measures to identify anomalies or risk signs much more quickly. Advanced data systems, for example, include AI-driven dashboards that combine data from several sources (e.g., lab findings, electronic patient-reported outcomes, electronic health records) and promptly identify outliers or protocol violations. For instance, Medidata's AI Intelligent Trials technology improves sponsors' capacity to predict enrollment and results by using predictive modeling to real-time trial performance parameters. Data quality and site risk are regularly scored by AI-enabled risk-based monitoring (RBM) technologies, which notify monitors of high-risk trends (such clusters of missing data or safety alerts) as soon as they appear [11, 12]. Because of this real-time monitoring, there is less need for thorough source-data verification at each location, concentrating human effort where AI can identify serious problems.

4.3.3 Remote Patient Supervision and Decentralized Trial Monitoring

Utilizing this real-time data requires the use of AI and machine learning. Compared to manual inspection, automated algorithms can continuously examine incoming measures to identify anomalies or risk signs much more quickly. Advanced data systems, for example, include AI-driven dashboards that combine data from several sources (e.g., lab findings, electronic patient-reported outcomes, electronic health records) and promptly identify outliers or protocol violations. For instance, Medidata's AI Intelligent Trials technology improves sponsors' capacity to predict enrollment and results by using predictive modeling to real-time trial performance parameters. Data quality and site risk are regularly scored by AI-enabled risk-based monitoring (RBM) technologies, which notify monitors of high-risk trends (such clusters of missing data or safety alerts) as soon as they appear [11, 12]. Because of this real-time monitoring, there is less need for thorough source-data verification at each location, concentrating human effort where AI can identify serious problems.

4.3.4 Safety, Efficacy, and Dynamic AI Systems

These methods of ongoing monitoring enhance the assurance of efficacy and safety. From a safety perspective, AI can quickly compile and evaluate reports of adverse events, changes in vital signs, or lab trends for every participant. For instance, real-time signal detection algorithms may identify an unanticipated pattern of elevated liver enzymes in a treatment arm, allowing researchers to modify dosage before significant toxicity occurs. Real-time analytics in efficacy analysis enable adaptive decisions: a trial can be changed or stopped sooner if interim data (such as biomarker responses) suggest that it is unlikely to reach its endpoint. On the other hand, enrollment might be increased if early efficacy signals are very robust. All things considered, AI lowers error and speeds up trial decision-making by "automating data gathering, checking data quality, and evaluating big datasets" in real-time.

In fact, contemporary AI systems in healthcare are rarely truly static. As Reddy et al. describe, a dynamic AI framework continuously ingests feedback and data post-deployment, adjusting model parameters to improve performance [13]. Figure 4.1 illustrates this concept: the traditional "train-then-freeze" approach (Fig. 4.1a) gives way to an adaptive system (Fig. 4.1b) where AI learns from incoming clinical data. Such adaptability is critical for real-time monitoring scenarios. For example, an AI-driven safety monitor might use reinforcement learning—analogous to the RLHF (reinforcement learning from human feedback) in large language models—to recalibrate alert thresholds as more safety

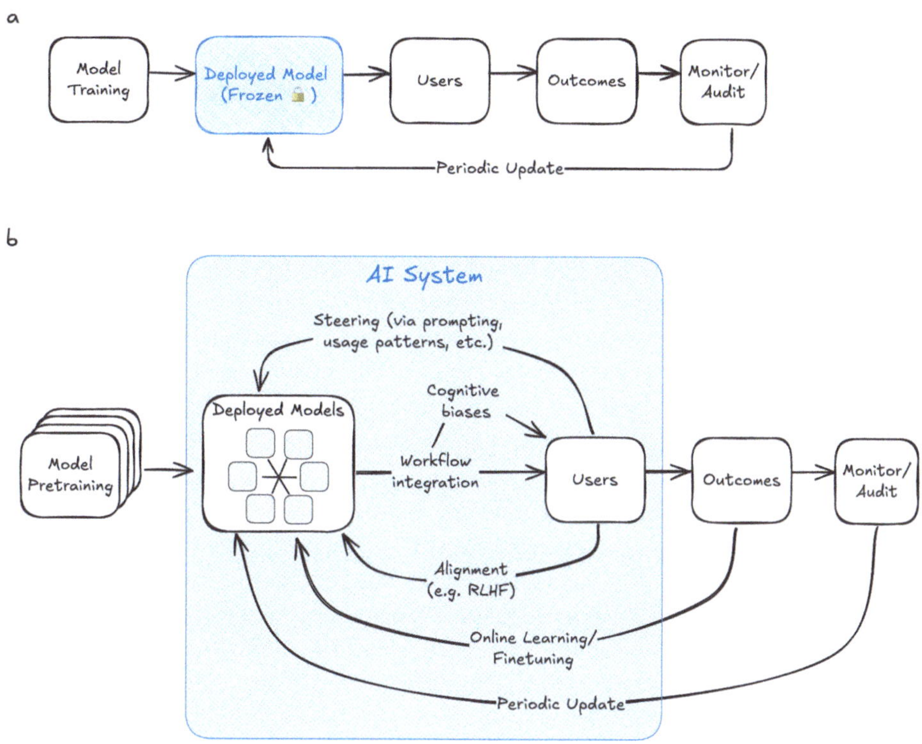

Fig. 4.1 Linear vs. dynamic AI deployment models. In the linear model (**a**), an AI model is trained and then deployed with fixed parameters, whereas in the dynamic model (**b**) the model continues to update from new data and user feedback

data arrive [13]. This ensures that the monitoring system itself improves over time rather than remaining rigid, thereby enhancing the trial's responsiveness to evolving patient information.

4.3.5 Infrastructure, Regulatory Support, and Future Outlook

Implementing real-time AI monitoring also necessitates robust data infrastructure. Electronic data capture (EDC) systems and clinical data platforms now support continuous integration of site, lab, imaging, and patient data. Advanced platforms (often cloud-based) can run AI analyses on these data in real time, generating live dashboards for trial sponsors and data monitoring committees. For example, Medidata Rave and similar systems use AI to automate query resolution; they can detect anomalous data entries immediately and notify sites to verify them. The result is a trial in which the data lifecycle is largely automated: data flow seamlessly from patients to analysis, with AI constantly "cleaning" and interpreting the data stream. As one review notes, AI can "automatically fill out the required analysis report" by feeding processed data into downstream systems, thereby saving time and reducing human error [12].

Crucially, regulators and sponsors are embracing these innovations. FDA and EMA guidance now encourage risk-based and remote monitoring strategies, which are naturally supported by AI. For example, recent FDA recommendations explicitly allow for telemedicine and wearable endpoints in trials, and novel AI-based predictors are being explored as trial endpoints. While a standardized regulatory framework for AI in research is still emerging, the emphasis is on ensuring trustworthy AI, i.e., validated algorithms, audit trails, and patient privacy safeguards. According to Reddy et al., the EU's proposed Artificial Intelligence Act categorizes high-risk medical AI (including trial oversight tools) under strict requirements. This means that any real-time monitoring AI must undergo rigorous validation, but once approved, it offers unparalleled continuity of oversight. Early adopters have reported tangible benefits: continuous monitoring "not only protects participants but also enhances the overall credibility of the trial" [14]. By catching data issues or safety signals early, AI-assisted monitoring can shorten trial timelines, reduce the number of required on-site audits, and ultimately speed up development of new therapies.

In summary, real-time data analysis and monitoring in clinical trials leverage AI to transform static trials into dynamic, continuously optimized studies. Through wearables, EHR integration, and smart analytics, investigators maintain a 24/7 view of trial conduct. AI algorithms play multiple roles: they detect outliers in the data, verify data quality on entry, predict patient non-compliance, and even suggest amendments to trial conduct in response to emerging patterns. This real-time vigilance can improve patient safety, ensure protocol fidelity, and accelerate decision-making—all of which make trials more efficient and effective [12].

4.4 Case Examples of AI-Supported Clinical Trials

4.4.1 AI for Patient Matching and Recruitment

The practical impact of AI in trials is best illustrated by real-world case studies. These examples span the trial spectrum—from patient recruitment to treatment selection—demonstrating how AI tools have already begun to change trial outcomes. One of the earliest successes involved AI-driven patient matching. Mayo Clinic partnered with IBM Watson Health to use natural language processing for trial enrollment. In a notable pilot, Watson for Clinical Trial Matching scanned thousands of patient records (clinical notes, lab reports, pathology) to identify eligible candidates for breast cancer trials. The result was striking within 11 months of deployment; Mayo Clinic saw an 80% increase in trial enrollment compared to manual matching methods [15]. Patients who would have fallen through the cracks were flagged as matches, and screening time per patient fell substantially. According to Mayo oncologist Dr. Tufia Haddad, this "enabled all patients to be screened for all available trial opportunities," greatly improving the pace of breast cancer studies.

This case shows AI's utility in the screening phase: by automating pattern recognition in medical data, AI can rapidly connect more patients with appropriate trials, addressing a common bottleneck in clinical research.

4.4.2 Large Language Models (LLMs) for Trial Eligibility Screening

More recently, AI has entered actual trial protocols. In 2024, NIH researchers published TrialGPT, a patient-to-trial matching system using large language models. TrialGPT uses an LLM to filter and rank trials for a given patient description. In tests on synthetic data, it recalled over 90% of relevant trials while reducing the initial candidate set by 94%. Crucially, when clinicians compared TrialGPT's eligibility predictions to expert review, the AI achieved 87.3% accuracy, nearly matching human performance. A user study even showed TrialGPT could cut screening time by 42.6%. In practice, this means a patient's chart could be algorithmically scanned against thousands of criteria in seconds, rather than requiring days of manual chart review. TrialGPT is illustrative of a broader trend: modern LLMs and AI systems are being trained to understand unstructured medical information, greatly speeding up the matching of patients to existing trials. As the study reports, such AI frameworks promise "promising opportunities for patient-to-trial matching" and could power future trial-matching platforms [16].

4.4.3 Precision Medicine Trials Using AI-Driven Treatment Selection (EXALT-1)

Another domain is **precision medicine** within trials. Exscientia and collaborators conducted a basket trial (EXALT-1) in aggressive hematological cancers using an AI-driven functional precision medicine platform. Instead of relying only on genetic biomarkers, this platform tested patients' tumor cells against a panel of drugs in vitro and used AI to predict the optimal therapy for each patient. In the EXALT-1 trial (published in *Cancer Discovery*), patients treated according to the AI platform's recommendations experienced significantly better outcomes. Overall, 54% of patients showed a greater than 1.3-fold increase in progression-free survival (PFS) over their prior therapy. Moreover, 40% of those responders had "exceptional" responses—PFS more than three times longer than expected. These results suggest that AI-enabled decision tools can meaningfully improve trial efficacy by personalizing treatment. As Exscientia's co-inventor put it, their AI system "provides prediction of a patient's response prior to deciding on a course of therapy," something genetic tests alone cannot do. Thus, EXALT-1 is a landmark example of an AI-assisted trial design: the study adapted treatment regimens based on real-time single-cell analyses, guided by machine learning, and demonstrated improved clinical benefit in a prospective setting [17].

4.4.4 AI in Diagnostic Imaging: The SMART Fracture Trial

AI has also been applied to image-based and diagnostic trials. Consider the ongoing "SMART Fracture Trial" in emergency medicine. This international randomized study is evaluating whether an **AI-assisted radiology tool** can detect bone fractures more quickly and accurately than standard radiologist interpretation. Patients are randomized to routine X-ray review or review augmented by an FDA-cleared AI system that highlights potential fractures on the image (Aidoc or Gleamer software). The trial's primary endpoints include diagnostic accuracy and time to diagnosis. By designing this prospective trial, the investigators are rigorously testing an AI device within the context of routine care. The stated goal is to quantify real-world benefits of AI—for example, whether AI assistance "expedites the process of diagnosing broken bones" or "reduces healthcare costs" through efficiency. This approach—embedding AI tools into live clinical workflows and measuring outcomes—exemplifies how AI trials can be structured. Initial expectations are that if the AI proves faster or more precise, it could lead to changes in emergency care protocols. Similar efforts are underway for other AI diagnostics; for instance, trials are registered to validate AI systems in dermatology, cardiology imaging, and more [18].

4.4.5 AI Tools for Patient Adherence and Engagement

Patient adherence and engagement are another area for AI intervention. Digital health companies have introduced AI-driven apps to boost compliance in trials. One example is a mobile platform (formerly called Pillsy, now known as Health) that reminds patients to take medications, provides instructional videos, and uses a smart pill bottle to track dosing. Such apps use AI to personalize reminders and interpret adherence data in real time, alerting both patient and study staff if doses are missed [12]. These tools are often tested in clinical studies to see if they can improve medication adherence and clinical outcomes. For example, an AI coach might adjust its communication style based on a patient's reported side effects, thereby maintaining engagement. Although still emerging, these AI engagement tools are being incorporated into larger trial designs to see if they can reduce dropout rates and ensure data completeness.

4.4.6 In Silico and Virtual Trial Enhancements with AI

Finally, AI can simulate or augment trial arms using historical data. Though not a human trial example per se, in silico trials use AI and computational models to predict outcomes of control groups. A recent analysis in oncology suggested that machine learning models could generate a "virtual control arm" from real-world data, potentially reducing the number of patients needed on placebo or standard therapy. Other exploratory studies have used generative AI to refine trial inclusion criteria by mining vast databases of prior trials and patient records to identify the most informative cohort. These cutting-edge approaches are still experimental, but they indicate future directions: AI may one day be power *adaptive* trials that evolve as results come in or even enable entirely virtual trials for certain questions.

In summary, the cases above illustrate AI's growing role across the clinical trial lifecycle. From patient recruitment (Mayo Watson, TrialGPT) to treatment optimization (Exscientia's precision medicine) and outcome monitoring (AI diagnostic aids, adherence apps), AI-enabled approaches are already being validated in prospective studies. These examples underscore the global impact of AI on trials: by automating complex tasks and extracting insights from data in real time, AI can make trials faster, smarter, and more patient centered. The collective experience suggests that AI-supported trials are not just a future promise but a current reality, yielding measurable improvements in efficiency and efficacy when thoughtfully deployed [16–18].

References

1. Zhang B, Zhang L, Chen Q, et al. Harnessing artificial intelligence to improve clinical trial design. Commun Med. 2023;3:191. https://doi.org/10.1038/s43856-023-00425-3.
2. Birkenbihl C, de Jong J, Yalchyk I, Fröhlich H. Deep learning-based patient stratification for prognostic enrichment of clinical dementia trials. Brain Commun. 2024;6(6):fcae445. https://doi.org/10.1093/braincomms/fcae445.
3. Schwager E, Jansson K, Rahman A, Schiffer S, Chang Y, Boverman G, Gross B, Xu-Wilson M, Boehme P, Truebel H, Frassica JJ. Utilizing machine learning to improve clinical trial design for acute respiratory distress syndrome. NPJ Digit Med. 2021;4(1):133. https://doi.org/10.1038/s41746-021-00505-5.
4. Oikonomou EK, Thangaraj PM, Bhatt DL, et al. An explainable machine learning-based phenomapping strategy for adaptive predictive enrichment in randomized clinical trials. NPJ Digit Med. 2023;6:217. https://doi.org/10.1038/s41746-023-00963-z.
5. Pallmann P, Bedding AW, Choodari-Oskooei B, et al. Adaptive designs in clinical trials: why use them, and how to run and report them. BMC Med. 2018;16:29. https://doi.org/10.1186/s12916-018-1017-7.
6. Azenkot T, Rivera DR, Stewart MD, Patel SP. Artificial intelligence and machine learning innovations to improve design and representativeness in oncology clinical trials. JCO Oncol Pract. 2025;21(Suppl):e473590. https://doi.org/10.1200/edbk-25-473590.
7. Lu X, Yang C, Liang L, Hu G, Zhong Z, Jiang Z. Artificial intelligence for optimizing recruitment and retention in clinical trials: a scoping review. J Am Med Inform Assoc. 2024;31(11):2749–59. https://doi.org/10.1093/jamia/ocae243.
8. Jayaraman P, Desman J, Sabounchi M, et al. A primer on reinforcement learning in medicine for clinicians. NPJ Digit Med. 2024;7:337. https://doi.org/10.1038/s41746-024-01316-0.
9. Zhao Y, Kosorok MR, Zeng D. Reinforcement learning design for cancer clinical trials. Stat Med. 2009;28(26):3294–315. https://doi.org/10.1002/sim.3720.
10. Kaylor A. How digital twins are reshaping clinical trials. Pharm Life Sci 2025 May 8. https://www.techtarget.com/pharmalifesciences/feature/How-digital-twins-are-reshaping-clinical-trials. Accessed 28 Jun 2025.

11. Shajari S, Kuruvinashetti K, Komeili A, Sundararaj U. The emergence of AI-based wearable sensors for digital health technology: a review. Sensors (Basel). 2023;23(23):9498. https://doi.org/10.3390/s23239498.
12. Chopra H, Annu SDK, Munjal K, Priyanka DK, Emran TB. Revolutionizing clinical trials: the role of AI in accelerating medical breakthroughs. Int J Surg. 2023;109(12):4211–20. https://doi.org/10.1097/JS9.0000000000000705.
13. Rosenthal JT, Beecy A, Sabuncu MR. Rethinking clinical trials for medical AI with dynamic deployments of adaptive systems. NPJ Digit Med. 2025;8:252. https://doi.org/10.1038/s41746-025-01674-3.
14. Young M. Continuous monitoring in clinical trials: enhancing safety and efficacy. Lindus Health [blog] 2025 Jun 13. https://www.lindushealth.com/blog/continuous-monitoring-in-clinical-trials-enhancing-safety-and-efficacy. Accessed 28 Jun 2025.
15. Kaylor A. Mayo Clinic finds 80% increase in clinical trial enrollment with IBM Watson. Pharm Life Sci. 2018 Mar 21. https://subjectwell.com/mayo-clinic-increase-clinical-trial-enrollment-ibm-watson/. Accessed 28 Jun 2025.
16. Jin Q, Wang Z, Floudas CS, et al. Matching patients to clinical trials with large language models. Nat Commun. 2024;15:9074. https://doi.org/10.1038/s41467-024-53081-z.
17. Exscientia. Publication of EXALT-1 trial in *cancer discovery* demonstrates first AI-supported functional precision medicine platform to improve cancer treatment outcomes. Press release 11 Oct 2021.
18. Salzburger Landeskliniken Betriebs gmbH. Assessing AI-Supported Fracture Detection in Emergency Care Units. ClinicalTrials.gov. Identifier: NCT06754137. Study start: 31 Mar 2025. Recruiting. https://clinicaltrials.gov/study/NCT06754137. Accessed 28 Jun 2025.

AI Drug Repurposing and Personalized Medicine

5

Drug repurposing, also known as drug repositioning, represents a transformative strategy within modern biopharma. This approach focuses on identifying novel therapeutic applications for pharmaceutical compounds that have already received regulatory approval or have undergone extensive preclinical and clinical investigation for other indications [1]. By leveraging existing safety and pharmacological data, drug repurposing significantly accelerates development timelines and mitigates the substantial financial risks typically associated with the traditional drug discovery process [1]. Historically, this process was often serendipitous; however, the advent of artificial intelligence (AI) has fundamentally reshaped it, transforming it into a systematic, efficient, and highly cost-effective endeavor [1].

Concurrently, personalized medicine, often referred to as precision medicine, signifies a profound paradigm shift in healthcare delivery. Departing from the conventional "one-size-fits-all" models, personalized medicine is dedicated to tailoring medical treatments, diagnostics, and overall healthcare strategies to align with an individual patient's unique genetic makeup, environmental exposures, lifestyle factors, and comprehensive medical history [2]. This bespoke approach is paramount for enhancing treatment efficacy, optimizing clinical outcomes, bolstering patient safety, and fostering greater patient engagement and adherence to therapeutic regimens [2]. The imperative for such tailored interventions arises from the recognition that a treatment beneficial for one patient could be ineffective or even detrimental to another, owing to inherent inter-individual variations [2].

Artificial intelligence has rapidly emerged as an indispensable tool in both drug repurpose and personalized medicine. By effectively harnessing vast and diverse datasets including electronic health records (EHRs), genomic sequences, proteomic profiles, data from wearable devices, and real-time clinical input, AI algorithms can systematically

K. Shaikh et al., *Artificial Intelligence in Drug Discovery and Development*,
Synthesis Lectures on Engineering, Science, and Technology,
https://doi.org/10.1007/978-3-032-10277-5_5

mine, predict, and validate new drug disease relationships. These capabilities extend to identifying intricate patterns, forecasting individual disease risks, and recommending highly personalized therapeutic strategies [1]. This integration of AI promises to accelerate drug discovery and development, enhancing diagnostic accuracy, optimizing treatment plans, and ultimately lead to improved patient outcomes [3]. It has greater operational efficiencies across the biopharmaceutical and broader healthcare sectors [3].

This chapter provides an in-depth explanation of the specific algorithmic approaches employed in AI-driven drug repurposing, the intricate mechanisms by which genomic profiling and multi-omics data are integrated with AI for personalized treatment alignment, the unique and critical applications of AI in addressing the formidable challenges posed by rare an orphan diseases, and the crucial ethical and regulatory considerations that are indispensable for the responsible, equitable, and effective deployment of AI in these rapidly evolving medical domains.

5.1 Algorithms for Drug Repurposing

AI-driven drug repurposing involves the systematic application of AI, particularly machine learning (ML) and deep learning (DL), to discover new therapeutic uses for existing, approved, or extensively studied drugs. This paradigm shift transforms drug discovery from a laborious, often serendipitous, and high-risk process into a highly efficient, cost-effective, and data-driven strategy [1]. The profound significance of this approach lies in its ability to drastically shorten traditional drug development timelines, potentially reducing them from 10–15 years to as little as 3–6 years by leveraging existing safety data and pharmacological information [1]. This also translates to significantly reduced financial investment and low risk, as AI-based repurposing minimizes the financial burden and increases the probability of successful market authorization by focusing on compounds with established safety profiles [1]. AI algorithms can screen thousands of compounds within hours, a task that would conventionally take years, thereby accelerating lead identification and optimizing research and development (R&D) budgets [1].

The application of AI in drug repurposing primarily leverages machine learning and deep learning models. These models are specifically designed to process large quantities of diverse data, encompassing genomic, proteomic, and clinical information, to identify complex patterns that can predict novel drug-disease relationships [1]. The common techniques and their applications in this domain are as follows:

- **Neural Networks (NNs)/Deep Neural Networks (DNNs):** These models are highly effective at analyzing complex, multidimensional data. For instance, encoder-decoder architectures with DNNs are designed to predict binding affinity scores, which are critical for evaluating how effectively a drug molecule interacts with its target protein. These models learn from extensive historical clinical data and large semantic knowledge graphs [1].

- **Support Vector Machines (SVMs):** As supervised learning models, SVMs are employed to process and analyze labeled data. They are trained to identify and construct drug target association patterns, enabling the prediction of potential novel target associations [4].
- **Random Forests:** This is another widely used supervised learning model, valued for its ability to model complex, nonlinear relationships between molecular structure and biological activity. This contributes to more sophisticated, data-driven drug design and prediction [1].
- **Graph Neural Networks (GNNs):** GNNs are particularly powerful for exploiting the interconnected nature of biological data. They can process heterogeneous biomedical graphs that include genes, proteins, and drugs, facilitating the prediction of multi-target effects. An example is DeepDrug, which uses an expert-led directed GNN to identify promising drug combinations for diseases like Alzheimer's. GNN excel is leveraging knowledge graphs (KGs) for drug discovery, demonstrating strong capabilities in link prediction and capturing intricate biological relationships [1].
- **Generative Adversarial Networks (GANs):** GANs represent a class of machine learning frameworks comprising a generator and a discriminator neural network. These are trained adversarially to generate new data samples that are like a given dataset. They hold immense potential in drug repurposing due to their ability to generate novel molecular structures, predict drug interactions, and optimize the pharmacokinetic properties of existing drugs [4].

In addition to these specific algorithms, AI-drive drug repurposing broadly utilizes different learning paradigms:

- **Similarity-Based Approaches:** These are among the most popular AI methods in drug repurposing, frequently employing supervised learning models. They operate on the principle of identifying potential therapeutic targets or new indications based on structural, functional, or phenotypic similarities between drugs, diseases, or targets [4].
- **Supervised Learning Models:** These models are trained on labeled datasets, meaning the input data is paired with corresponding known outputs. They learn to identify patterns and construct predictive models for drug-target associations, enabling the prediction of novel target interactions. Examples include linear regression, logistic regression, and Boltzmann networks [4].
- **Unsupervised Learning Models:** Unlike supervised methods, these models work with unlabeled data. Their primary use in drug repurposing is to extract representative attributes and hidden patterns from raw drug features, allowing for the inference of potential targets or drug uses based on inherent data similarities. K-means clustering and principal component analysis (PCA) are typical examples [4].

5.1.1 Strengths of AI in Accelerating Drug Repurposing

The integration of AI offers several compelling advantages that significantly accelerate drug repurposing efforts:

- **Shortened Development Timelines:** AI drastically reduces the extensive timeframes (typically 10–15 years) associated with traditional drug discovery. By leveraging existing safety data and pharmacological information, AI algorithms can screen thousands of compounds within hours, a process that might otherwise take years using conventional experimental methods, thereby accelerating lead identification and preclinical stages [1].
- **Reduced Financial Investment and Lower Risk:** The cost of developing a new chemical entity can exceed billions of dollars, and clinical trial failure rates are notoriously high. AI-based repurpose minimizes financial risk by focusing on compounds that have already passed initial safety testing. Predictive models that combine binding affinity scores and pharmacokinetic properties ensure that only the most promising candidates are advanced, optimizing R&D budgets and reducing overall investment risk [1].
- **Data-Driven Decision-Making:** AI enhances decision accuracy by integrating multiple, heterogeneous data sources including clinical trial data, gene-disease associations, molecular interaction networks, unstructured data from patents, scientific literature, and electronics health records (EHRs). This allows for faster analysis than human experts could manage manually, reducing human error and enabling a more objective evaluation of drug efficacy and safety profiles [1].
- **Scalability and High-Throughput Screening:** AI systems can evaluate millions of virtual compounds in a fraction of the time, offering massive scalability that traditional early-phase development cannot match. This high-throughput capability drastically boosts preclinical speed by predicting toxicity, effectiveness, and pharmacokinetics before laboratory synthesis [1].
- **Mechanism Elucidation:** Beyond merely identifying candidates, AI provides deeper insights into complex molecular mechanisms underlying drug disease relationships that were previously too intricate to resolve through conventional methods [1].

5.1.2 Limitations of Current AI Algorithms

Despite these strengths, current AI algorithms in drug repurposing face several limitations:

- **Data Quality and Availability:** A fundamental limitation is the reliance on high-quality, vast, and diverse datasets. The availability, completeness, and representativeness of data can significantly hinder the accuracy and reliability of AI predictions. In complete biomedical knowledge graphs, for instance, pose a key challenge [5].

- **Interpretability/Explainability:** Many advanced AI models, particularly deep learning architectures, often operate as "black boxes," making it challenging to understand the underlying reasoning for their predictions. This lack of interpretability can impede trust and adoption among clinicians and researchers who require transparent insights for critical decision-making [6].
- **Computational Costs:** While powerful, certain algorithms like graph neural networks can incur substantial computational costs when applied to extremely large-scale knowledge graphs, limiting their practical deployment in some contexts [5].
- **Generalizability:** A significant drawback for some AI models, including GNNs, is their critical failure to generalize effectively to unseen entities or novel scenarios. This is a particular concern in drug discovery, where new drugs, diseases, and biological interactions are continuously emerging [5].

5.1.3 Broader Implication of AI in Drug Repurposing

The integration of AI into drug repurposing signifies a fundamental methodological shift within pharmaceutical research and development. This transition moves from relying on chance observations or exhaustive, undirected screening to a highly predictive, data-driven, and systematic approach [1]. This change minimizes the element of "luck" and significantly increases the probability of identifying high confidence drug candidates earlier in the pipeline, by leveraging AI's ability to discern complex, non-obvious patterns in vast datasets. This transformation has profound implications for the entire pharmaceutical R&D landscape. It suggests a future where investment shifts from broad, undirected experimental screening to more targeted computationally guided hypothesis generation and validation. This could lead to a higher return on investment for R&D efforts, accelerate the market entry of all new therapies (not just repurposed ones, as the underlying AI methodologies are generalizable), and fundamentally alter the economic models and risk profiles associated with pharmaceutical innovation. The industry may increasingly pivot toward building robust AI capabilities and data infrastructures as core competencies.

Furthermore, the effectiveness and reliability of advanced AI algorithms, such as GNNs and GANs, are intrinsically linked to the quality, completeness, representativeness, and accessibility of the data on which they are trained. While algorithms are becoming increasingly sophisticated, their practical limitations, such as generalization failures or training instabilities, often stem from inherent challenges in real-world biological data, including missing values, batch effects, or biases, or the difficulty of optimizing complex models on imperfect data [5]. The promise of "high-precision and efficient identification" [4] is therefore critically contingent on overcoming these pervasive data-centric hurdles. This interdependence highlights a crucial feedback loop continuous advancements in AI algorithms necessitate even higher quality, more comprehensive, and better-structured data. This, in turn, drives an urgent need for improved data collection methodologies, standardization efforts, and sophisticated data integration strategies across the biomedical research ecosystem.

From a regulatory perspective, this implies that agencies like the FDA and EMA will increasingly scrutinize not just the AI algorithms themselves but also the provenance, quality, and bias mitigation strategies of the training dataset as a core component of their review and approval processes [7]. Future success in AI-driven drug repurposing will thus depend as much on establishing robust data governance frameworks and collaborative data-sharing initiatives as it will on developing novel algorithmic architectures.

5.1.4 Practical Examples of Drug Repurposing

As we know that, drug repositioning (or repurposing) aims to find new uses for existing drugs. AI algorithms can achieve this by identifying similarities between diseases, drugs, or drug-disease interactions from various data sources. There are few conceptual approaches with codes that are used in this purpose.

- **Similarity-based methods:** Cluster drugs or diseases based on various features (e.g., chemical structure, gene expression profiles, side effects). If a known drug treats a disease, similar drugs might treat similar diseases.

```
import pandas as pd
from sklearn.cluster import KMeans
from sklearn.preprocessing import StandardScaler
from sklearn.metrics.pairwise import cosine_similarity
import numpy as np

# --- 1. Simulate Data ---
# Let's imagine we have gene expression data for various diseases and drugs
# For simplicity, gene expression is represented as numerical vectors.
# In reality, this would come from RNA-seq or microarray data.

# Disease Gene Expression Profiles (e.g., differential expression of 100 genes)
# Disease A, B, C have known drugs. Disease X is a new disease.
data_diseases = {
    'Disease': ['DiseaseA', 'DiseaseB', 'DiseaseC', 'DiseaseX'],
    'Gene_Exp_1': [0.5, 0.6, 0.4, 0.55],
    'Gene_Exp_2': [0.8, 0.7, 0.9, 0.75],
    'Gene_Exp_3': [0.2, 0.3, 0.1, 0.25],
    # ... up to Gene_Exp_100 (truncated for brevity)
    'Gene_Exp_N': [0.7, 0.8, 0.6, 0.72],
}
df_diseases = pd.DataFrame(data_diseases)

# Known Drug-Disease Associations
known_drug_disease = {
    'DiseaseA': ['Drug1', 'Drug2'],
    'DiseaseB': ['Drug3'],
    'DiseaseC': ['Drug4', 'Drug5'],
}

print("--- Simulated Disease Gene Expression Data ---")
print(df_diseases.head())
print("\n--- Known Drug-Disease Associations ---")
for disease, drugs in known_drug_disease.items():
    print(f"{disease}: {', '.join(drugs)}")

# --- 2. Preprocess Data ---
# Features for clustering are the gene expression columns
X = df_diseases.drop('Disease', axis=1)

# Scale the features
scaler = StandardScaler()
X_scaled = scaler.fit_transform(X)

# --- 3. Cluster Diseases ---
# Use KMeans to group diseases based on similarity of gene expression.
# The number of clusters (n_clusters) would typically be determined by
# methods like the elbow method or domain knowledge.
n_clusters = 3 # Example number of clusters
kmeans = KMeans(n_clusters=n_clusters, random_state=42, n_init=10)
df_diseases['Cluster'] = kmeans.fit_predict(X_scaled)

print("\n--- Diseases with Assigned Clusters ---")
print(df_diseases[['Disease', 'Cluster']])

# --- 4. Identify Potential Repositioning for 'DiseaseX' ---
target_disease_name = 'DiseaseX'
target_disease_cluster = df_diseases[df_diseases['Disease'] ==
target_disease_name]['Cluster'].iloc[0]

# Find diseases in the same cluster as DiseaseX (excluding DiseaseX itself)
similar_diseases = df_diseases[
    (df_diseases['Cluster'] == target_disease_cluster) &
    (df_diseases['Disease'] != target_disease_name)
]['Disease'].tolist()

print(f"\n'{target_disease_name}' is in Cluster {target_disease_cluster}.")
print(f"Diseases in the same cluster: {', '.join(similar_diseases)}")

# Collect drugs from similar diseases that have known treatments
repositioned_drugs = set()
for disease in similar_diseases:
    if disease in known_drug_disease:
        repositioned_drugs.update(known_drug_disease[disease])

if repositioned_drugs:
    print(f"\nSuggested drugs for '{target_disease_name}' based on repositioning: {',
'.join(repositioned_drugs)}")
else:
    print(f"\nNo direct drug repositioning suggestions for '{target_disease_name}' found in its
cluster.")
```

An example is **a simple clustering algorithm that groups diseases based on their gene expression profiles and then suggests drugs for a new disease if it clusters with diseases that have known drug treatments.** In this conceptual code, we create dummy DataFrames for disease gene expression and known drug-disease associations. In real applications, there would be large, complex datasets from public databases (e.g., GEO, CTD, DrugBank) or proprietary sources. StandardScaler is used to normalize gene expression data, which is crucial for distance-based algorithms like **KMeans**. Diseases are grouped into clusters based on their gene expression similarity. Diseases in the same cluster are assumed to share underlying biological mechanisms. If a new disease falls into a cluster with diseases that are already treated by certain drugs, those drugs become candidates for repositioning. The output of the code is as follows:

```
--- Simulated Disease Gene Expression Data ---
    Disease  Gene_Exp_1  Gene_Exp_2  Gene_Exp_3  Gene_Exp_N
0  DiseaseA        0.50        0.80        0.20        0.70
1  DiseaseB        0.60        0.70        0.30        0.80
2  DiseaseC        0.40        0.90        0.10        0.60
3  DiseaseX        0.55        0.75        0.25        0.72

--- Known Drug-Disease Associations ---
DiseaseA: Drug1, Drug2
DiseaseB: Drug3
DiseaseC: Drug4, Drug5

--- Diseases with Assigned Clusters ---
    Disease  Cluster
0  DiseaseA        2
1  DiseaseB        0
2  DiseaseC        1
3  DiseaseX        2

'DiseaseX' is in Cluster 2.
Diseases in the same cluster: DiseaseA

Suggested drugs for 'DiseaseX' based on repositioning: Drug2, Drug1
```

- **Network-based methods:** Network-based approaches model biological and chemical entities (drugs, proteins, genes, diseases) as nodes in a graph and their relationships (interactions, associations) as edges. Drug repositioning often involves finding new connections or patterns within this network. The conceptual approach includes the following: (a) using heterogeneous networks which combine different types of nodes and edges; (b) identifying paths between a drug and a disease through intermediate biological entities; (c) predicting the likelihood of a new edge (e.g., drug disease association) forming based on existing network structure; and (d) simulating information flow through the network to identify nodes strongly connected to a query node (e.g., finding diseases related to a drug).

The below example (in the given code) creates a small, artificial heterogeneous network of drugs, targets (proteins), and diseases. It then demonstrates how to find paths between a drug and a disease, suggesting a potential repositioning if a plausible path exists. In the code, we use the networkx library to create a Graph object. Nodes represent drugs, proteins, and diseases, and edges represent their known relationships. We add type attributes to nodes (e.g., "drug," "protein," "disease") and relation attributes to edges (e.g., "targets," "interacts_with," "associated_with"). This makes it a heterogeneous network. A basic visualization helps understand the network structure. The core of this example is finding all simple paths (no repeated nodes) between a given target_drug and target_disease. The cutoff parameter limits the maximum length of paths to consider, which is important in large networks to avoid computationally expensive searches and biologically less relevant long paths.

```
import networkx as nx
import matplotlib.pyplot as plt
import random

# --- 1. Create a Heterogeneous Network ---
G = nx.Graph()

# Add Nodes: Drugs, Proteins (Targets), Diseases
drugs = ['DrugA', 'DrugB', 'DrugC', 'DrugD']
proteins = ['Protein1', 'Protein2', 'Protein3', 'Protein4', 'Protein5']
diseases = ['DiseaseX', 'DiseaseY', 'DiseaseZ']

G.add_nodes_from(drugs, type='drug')
G.add_nodes_from(proteins, type='protein')
G.add_nodes_from(diseases, type='disease')

# Add Edges:
# Drug-Protein interactions (known targets)
G.add_edge('DrugA', 'Protein1', relation='targets')
G.add_edge('DrugA', 'Protein2', relation='targets')
G.add_edge('DrugB', 'Protein2', relation='targets')
G.add_edge('DrugC', 'Protein3', relation='targets')
G.add_edge('DrugD', 'Protein4', relation='targets') # DrugD targets Protein4

# Protein-Protein interactions (e.g., from PPI databases)
G.add_edge('Protein1', 'Protein3', relation='interacts_with')
G.add_edge('Protein2', 'Protein5', relation='interacts_with')
G.add_edge('Protein3', 'Protein4', relation='interacts_with') # Protein3 interacts
with Protein4

# Protein-Disease associations (e.g., genes/proteins implicated in disease)
G.add_edge('Protein1', 'DiseaseX', relation='associated_with')
G.add_edge('Protein3', 'DiseaseY', relation='associated_with')
G.add_edge('Protein4', 'DiseaseZ', relation='associated_with') # Protein4 associ-
ated with DiseaseY

print("--- Network Nodes and Edges ---")
print(f"Nodes: {G.nodes()}")
print(f"Edges: {G.edges()}")

# --- 2. Visualize the Network (Optional) ---
# Assign colors based on node type for better visualization
node_colors = []
for node in G.nodes():
    node_type = G.nodes[node]['type']
    if node_type == 'drug':
        node_colors.append('skyblue')
    elif node_type == 'protein':
        node_colors.append('lightcoral')
    elif node_type == 'disease':
        node_colors.append('lightgreen')

plt.figure(figsize=(10, 8))
pos = nx.spring_layout(G, k=0.5, iterations=50) # Layout for visualization
nx.draw_networkx_nodes(G, pos, node_color=node_colors, node_size=3000)
nx.draw_networkx_edges(G, pos, edge_color='gray', alpha=0.6)
nx.draw_networkx_labels(G, pos, font_size=10, font_weight='bold')
plt.title("Heterogeneous Drug-Protein-Disease Network")
plt.savefig('network_visualization.png')
plt.show()

# --- 3. Find Paths for Drug Repositioning ---
# Goal: Can DrugD be repositioned for DiseaseY?
target_drug = 'DrugD'
target_disease = 'DiseaseY'
print(f"\n--- Searching for repositioning paths from '{target_drug}' to '{tar-
get_disease}' ---")
```

```
# Find all simple paths between the drug and the disease
# max_length can be set to limit path complexity
all_paths = list(nx.all_simple_paths(G, source=target_drug, target=target_disease,
cutoff=3)) # Limit path length to 3 for simplicity

if all_paths:
    print(f"Found {len(all_paths)} potential repositioning paths:")
    for i, path in enumerate(all_paths):
        path_str = " -> ".join(path)
        print(f"Path {i+1}: {path_str}")
        # Interpret the path:
        # Example path: DrugD -> Protein4 -> DiseaseY
        # Interpretation: DrugD targets Protein4, and Protein4 is associated with
DiseaseY.
        # This suggests DrugD might be effective for DiseaseY.

        # Example path: DrugD -> Protein4 -> Protein3 -> DiseaseY
        # Interpretation: DrugD targets Protein4, Protein4 interacts with Protein3,
        # and Protein3 is associated with DiseaseY. More indirect, but still a
lead.

    # A more sophisticated approach would score paths based on edge types,
    # confidence of interactions, and path length.
else:
    print(f"No direct or indirect paths found between '{target_drug}' and
'{target_disease}' within cutoff.")

# Another example: DrugC to DiseaseX
target_drug_2 = 'DrugC'
target_disease_2 = 'DiseaseX'
print(f"\n--- Searching for repositioning paths from '{target_drug_2}' to
'{target_disease_2}' ---")
all_paths_2 = list(nx.all_simple_paths(G, source=target_drug_2,
target=target_disease_2, cutoff=3))

if all_paths_2:
    print(f"Found {len(all_paths_2)} potential repositioning paths:")
    for i, path in enumerate(all_paths_2):
        path_str = " -> ".join(path)
        print(f"Path {i+1}: {path_str}")
else:
    print(f"No direct or indirect paths found between '{target_drug_2}' and
'{target_disease_2}' within cutoff.")
```

Each path found represents a potential biological mechanism by which the drug could influence the disease (as shown in Fig. 5.1). For instance, DrugD - > Protein4 - > DiseaseY suggests that if DrugD targets Protein4 and Protein4 is involved in DiseaseY, then DrugD might be effective for DiseaseY. In real applications, these paths would be analyzed for their biological plausibility and strength.

- **Machine Learning/Deep Learning:** Train models to predict drug-disease associations based on feature vectors derived from various omics data, chemical structures, and clinical data. The code below describes a basic neural network to predict if a drug-disease pair is associated, based on simplified numerical features for both. Here, first

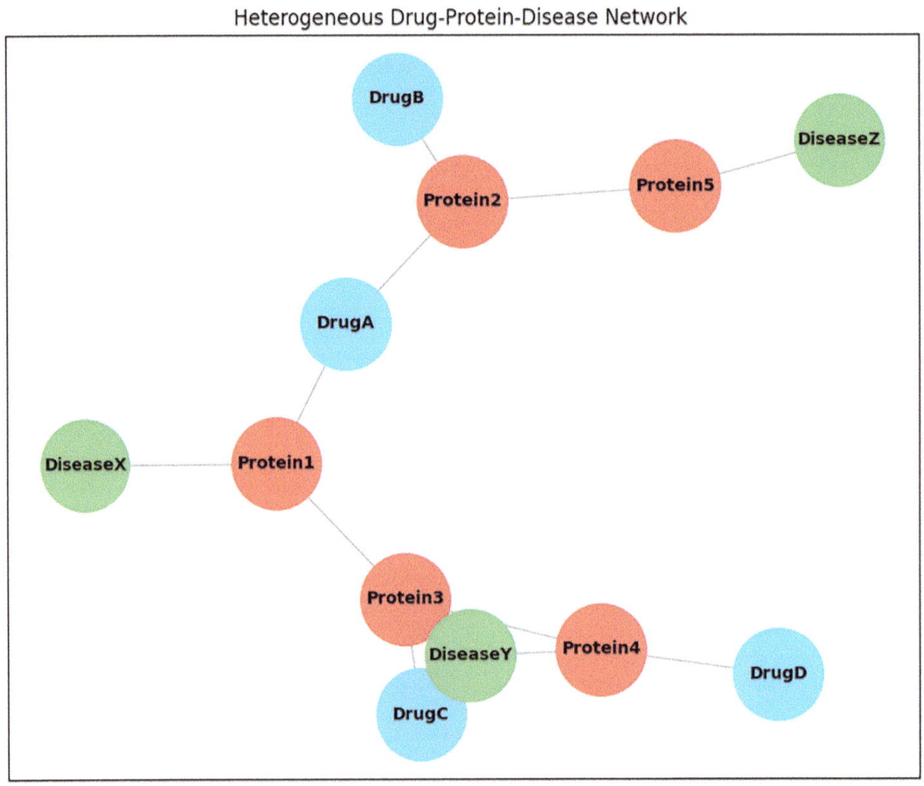

Fig. 5.1 Example of heterogeneous drug-protein-disease network

we generate random numerical features for drugs and diseases and combine them. A binary label (0 or 1) indicates whether a drug-disease pair is associated. In a real scenario, features would be carefully engineered from various data sources such as chemical properties, genomic data, and clinical trial outcomes.

```
import pandas as pd
import numpy as np
from sklearn.model_selection import train_test_split
from sklearn.preprocessing import StandardScaler
from tensorflow.keras.models import Sequential
from tensorflow.keras.layers import Dense, Dropout
from tensorflow.keras.optimizers import Adam
from sklearn.metrics import roc_auc_score, precision_recall_curve, auc
import matplotlib.pyplot as plt

# --- 1. Simulate Data ---
# Create synthetic features for drugs and diseases.
# In a real scenario, these would be derived from chemical structures,
# genomic data, etc.
num_samples = 50000
num_drug_features = 50
num_disease_features = 50

# Generate random features for drugs and diseases
np.random.seed(42)
drug_features = np.random.rand(num_samples, num_drug_features)
disease_features = np.random.rand(num_samples, num_disease_features)

# Combine drug and disease features into a single feature vector for each pair
X = np.hstack((drug_features, disease_features))

# Generate synthetic labels: 1 for associated, 0 for not associated
# Create a balanced dataset for demonstration
num_positive = num_samples // 2
num_negative = num_samples - num_positive
y = np.array([1] * num_positive + [0] * num_negative)
np.random.shuffle(y) # Shuffle labels to mix positive and negative samples

print("--- Simulated Drug-Disease Feature Data ---")
print(f"Shape of features (X): {X.shape}")
print(f"Shape of labels (y): {y.shape}")
print(f"Number of positive associations: {np.sum(y == 1)}")
print(f"Number of negative associations: {np.sum(y == 0)}")

# --- 2. Preprocess Data ---
# Split data into training and testing sets
X_train, X_test, y_train, y_test = train_test_split(X, y, test_size=0.2,
random_state=42, stratify=y)

# Scale features
scaler = StandardScaler()
X_train_scaled = scaler.fit_transform(X_train)
X_test_scaled = scaler.transform(X_test)

print("\n--- Data Split and Scaled ---")
print(f"X_train_scaled shape: {X_train_scaled.shape}")
print(f"X_test_scaled shape: {X_test_scaled.shape}")

# --- 3. Build a Simple Feed-Forward Neural Network Model ---
input_dim = X_train_scaled.shape[1] # Total number of features (drug_features +
disease_features)

model = Sequential([
    Dense(128, activation='relu', input_shape=(input_dim,)), # Input layer
    Dropout(0.3), # Dropout for regularization
    Dense(64, activation='relu'), # Hidden layer
    Dropout(0.3),
    Dense(32, activation='relu'), # Another hidden layer
    Dense(1, activation='sigmoid') # Output layer for binary classification
(sigmoid for probability)
])
```

```
# Compile the model
model.compile(optimizer=Adam(learning_rate=0.001),
              loss='binary_crossentropy', # Appropriate for binary classification
              metrics=['accuracy'])

model.summary()

# --- 4. Train the Model ---
print("\n--- Training the Neural Network ---")
history = model.fit(X_train_scaled, y_train,
                    epochs=20, # Number of training epochs
                    batch_size=32, # Number of samples per gradient update
                    validation_split=0.1, # Use 10% of training data for validation
                    verbose=1)

# --- 5. Evaluate the Model ---
loss, accuracy = model.evaluate(X_test_scaled, y_test, verbose=0)
print(f"\nTest Loss: {loss:.4f}")
print(f"Test Accuracy: {accuracy:.4f}")

# Predict probabilities on the test set
y_pred_proba = model.predict(X_test_scaled).ravel()

# Calculate ROC AUC score
roc_auc = roc_auc_score(y_test, y_pred_proba)
print(f"ROC AUC Score: {roc_auc:.4f}")

# Plot training history
plt.figure(figsize=(12, 5))
plt.subplot(1, 2, 1)
plt.plot(history.history['accuracy'], label='Train Accuracy')
plt.plot(history.history['val_accuracy'], label='Validation Accuracy')
plt.title('Model Accuracy')
plt.xlabel('Epoch')
plt.ylabel('Accuracy')
plt.legend()

plt.subplot(1, 2, 2)
plt.plot(history.history['loss'], label='Train Loss')
plt.plot(history.history['val_loss'], label='Validation Loss')
plt.title('Model Loss')
plt.xlabel('Epoch')
plt.ylabel('Loss')
plt.legend()
plt.show()


# --- 6. Make a Prediction for a New Drug-Disease Pair ---
# Simulate new drug and disease features
new_drug_features_single = np.random.rand(2, num_drug_features)
new_disease_features_single = np.random.rand(2, num_disease_features)
new_pair_features = np.hstack((new_drug_features_single,
new_disease_features_single))
print(new_pair_features)
# Scale the new features using the same scaler fitted on training data
new_pair_features_scaled = scaler.transform(new_pair_features)

predicted_probability = model.predict(new_pair_features_scaled)[0][0]

print(f"\n--- Prediction for a New Drug-Disease Pair ---")
print(f"Predicted probability of association: {predicted_probability:.4f}")
if predicted_probability > 0.5: # Using 0.5 as a simple threshold
    print("Prediction: This drug-disease pair is likely associated (potential
repositioning candidate).")
else:
    print("Prediction: This drug-disease pair is likely NOT associated.")
```

After that, data is split to evaluate the model's performance on unseen data. Stratify = y ensures that the proportion of positive and negative samples is maintained in both sets. Features are scaled to have zero mean and unit variance, which is crucial for neural networks to converge efficiently. A simple feed-forward neural network is constructed with multiple dense (fully connected) layers. Relu (rectified linear unit) is a common activation function for hidden layers. Dropout layers are added for regularization to prevent overfitting. The final dense layer has one neuron with a sigmoid activation function, outputting a probability between 0 and 1 for binary classification. The model is compiled with an Adam optimizer (a popular choice), binary_crossentropy loss (suitable for binary classification), and accuracy as a metric. The model is trained on the scaled training data. Epochs define the number of passes over the entire dataset, and batch_size determines how many samples are processed before updating the model weights. validation_split is used to monitor performance on a portion of the training data during training. The model's performance is evaluated on the unseen test set using loss, accuracy, and ROC AUC score (a common metric for imbalanced classification problems). Once trained, the model can predict the probability of association for new, unseen drug-disease pairs. The output of the code is as follows:

```
Test Loss: 0.7079
Test Accuracy: 0.4961
313/313 ━━━━━━━━━━━━━━━━━━━━ 0s 641us/step
ROC AUC Score: 0.4969

--- Prediction for a New Drug-Disease Pair ---
Predicted probability of association: 0.5885
Prediction: This drug-disease pair is likely associated (potential repositioning candidate).
```

5.2 Genomic Profiling and Treatment Alignment

Personalized medicine aims to deliver tailored medical treatments, diagnostics, and healthcare strategies that are customized to an individual's unique genetic makeup, lifestyle, and medical history, thereby moving beyond the traditional "one-size-fits-all" approach [2]. The foundation of personalized medicine lies in its ability to harness and analyze vast and diverse datasets. These include electronic health records (EHRs), comprehensive genomic sequences, data from wearable devices, and real-time clinical inputs [2]. By processing this rich information, AI algorithms can identify subtle patterns, predict individual disease risks, and recommend highly personalized therapeutic strategies that are optimized for each patient [2]. The imperative for tailoring treatments is underscored by the understanding that a therapeutic intervention beneficial for one patient might be ineffective or even harmful to another, owing to inherent inter-individual variations in genetic predispositions, environmental exposures, and lifestyle factors [2]. Personalized treatment aims to optimize clinical outcomes, avoid drugs or interventions unlikely to benefit a specific patient, enhance patient engagement and adherence, enable proactive health measures tailored to individual susceptibility, and ultimately lead to more cost effective and efficient healthcare [2].

5.2.1 The Role of Genomic Profiling and Multi-Omics Data

Genomic profiling involves comprehensive analysis of a patient's genetic data to predict their response to specific medications. This includes understanding genetic variations that influence drug metabolism, efficacy, and potential toxicity, as well as identifying genetic biomarkers crucial for disease diagnosis and treatment [8]. Multi-omics refers to the integrated analysis of high-throughput datasets that capture various molecular layers within biological systems. These layers provide a holistic view of cellular function and disease processes, encompassing [9]:

- **Genomics:** This provides information on an individual's genetic variation, such as single nucleotides polymorphisms (SNPs), insertions, deletions, and copy number variations [9].
- **Transcriptomics:** This involves data on gene expression, revealing which genes are active and to what extent [9].
- **Proteomics:** This is the analysis of protein levels, modifications, and interactions, which are the primary functional molecules in cells [9].
- **Metabolomics:** This characterizes small molecules metabolites, reflecting the downstream effects of genetic and environmental factors [9].
- **Epigenomics:** This is the study of epigenetic modifications (e.g., DNA methylation, histone modifications) that influence gene expression without altering the underlying DNA sequence [9].

By simultaneously probing these diverse biological aspects, multi-omics studies offer an unparalleled, holistic view of disease mechanisms, which is crucial for unraveling the complex, multifactorial nature of conditions such as cancer, rare genetic disorders, and autoimmune diseases [10].

5.2.2 Mechanisms of AI Integration for Treatment Alignment

AI plays a pivotal role in analyzing the vast and complex amounts of genetic and multi-omics data generated, processing intricate information, identifying subtle patterns, and making precise predictions about patient responses to medications [8]. Pharmacogenomics (PGx), a specialized field, investigates how an individual's genes affect their response to drugs. The integration of AI into PGx has opened new avenues for developing highly targeted treatment plans and significantly improving patient outcomes [8]. AI models analyze genomic data to identify genetic variants associated with both disease susceptibility and individual drug response [11]. AI-powered predictive models are capable of forecasting patient responses to various treatments based on their unique genomic and multi-omics profiles. This capability empowers healthcare professionals to develop highly personalized treatment strategies [8]. Key integration mechanisms for multi-omics data include:

- **Data Preprocessing and Normalization:** Before integration, rigorous data preprocessing and normalization are essential to mitigate technical biases and ensure comparability across heterogeneous omics datasets. This includes techniques for handling missing data, correcting batch effects that arise from different experimental setups, and scaling/transforming data to harmonize scales and distributions [9].
- **Dimensionality Reduction:** Preliminary feature selection or unsupervised learning techniques are often applied to reduce the complexity of high dimensional omics data.
- **Integration Stages:** Multi-omics data integration can be approached at different stages of the analysis pipeline [9]:
  - **Early Integration (Feature-Level Concatenation):** Raw or preprocessed features from different omics datasets are directly combined into a single, larger dataset before any downstream analysis.
  - **Intermediate Integration:** Omics-specific representations or embedding (lower-dimensional, meaningful summaries of each omics type) are first generated, and then these representations are fused.
  - **Late Integration (Decision-Level Fusion):** Independent models are trained on individual omics modality. Their predictions are then combined using ensemble techniques such as stacking, voting, or weighted averaging, leveraging the strengths of each modality's model while maintaining modularity.
- **Advanced Fusion Techniques:** Increasingly, sophisticated methods combine these paradigms with attention mechanisms and multi-task learning to optimize integration and enhance interpretability of the combined data.
- **Algorithm Examples:** Machine learning algorithms such as random forest, support vector machines (SVMs), and various deep learning architectures are extensively used for genomic data analysis [11]. Frameworks like MOGONET utilize graph convolutional networks (GCNs) for omics-specific learning and integrate these networks at the label space to improve classification performance in precision oncology [10].

A crucial aspect of practical implementation is the integration of AI algorithms with existing healthcare IT infrastructure. This includes electronic health records (EHRs) and clinical decision support systems (CDSSs), which enable healthcare professionals to access genomic data and AI-powered predictive models directly at the point of care, providing real-time guidance on treatment decisions [8].

5.2.3 Specific AI Applications in Personalized Medicine

AI applications are transforming treatment planning across various medical domains:

- **AI in Cancer Treatment Planning:** IBM Watson for Oncology exemplifies AI's application by analyzing patient medical records, pathology reports, and genomic data. It matches patient-specific tumor profiles with the latest clinical guidelines and research to identify targeted therapies and reduce treatment decision time, thereby improving patient care quality [2]. Furthermore, multi-omics integration coupled with AI has revolutionized cancer treatment by integrating genomic mutations (e.g., BRCA1/2), transcriptomic expression, and proteomic signaling pathways to guide the precision use of targeted therapies like PARP inhibitors. AI models can also predict chemotherapeutic resistance by analyzing epigenomic data [9].
- **Personalized Diabetes Management Using Continuous Glucose Monitoring (CGM):** AI-powered platforms process real-time data streamed from CGM devices. These platforms predict glucose fluctuations and recommend personalized insulin dosing or dietary adjustments based on an individual's metabolic responses. This leads to improved glycemic control and a reduced risk of hypoglycemia compared to standard protocols [2].
- **Personalized Mental Health Treatment:** AI analyses genetic clinical and behavioral patterns to predict treatment responses for mental health conditions. AI-driven biomarker analysis has been instrumental in developing personalized treatment plans for depression and schizophrenia, reducing the traditional trail-and-error prescribing approach [2].

5.2.4 Broader Implications of Genomic Profiling and Treatment Alignment

The true transformative power of AI in personalized medicine is not merely its ability to analyze vast and complex biological datasets. Rather, it lies in the capacity to translate that sophisticated analysis into clinically actionable insights that can be delivered directly at the point of care [8]. This requires seamless, bidirectional integration of AI models with existing healthcare IT infrastructure, such as EHRs and CDSSs, to provide timely, personalized recommendations to clinicians. Without this effective integration into clinical workflows, the insights generated by AI remain theoretical and fail to realize their full potential in improving patient outcomes. This implies a significant evolution in the role of clinicians, moving from solely interpreting disparate raw data to effectively leveraging AI-powered decision support systems as augmented intelligence. It also underscores the critical need for robust interoperability standards, secure data exchange protocols, and advanced IT infrastructure within healthcare systems to fully enable personalized medicine at scale. The success of AI in this domain hinges not just on algorithmic prowess but on effective human-AI collaboration and systemic integration, suggesting that healthcare institutions must invest heavily in both technological infrastructure and the training of their workforce to adapt to these new modalities of care delivery.

Moreover, the concept of "personalized" in medicine is continuously expanding and deepening. It has evolved beyond a primary focus on genomics to encompass a much broader, integrated spectrum of biological data, often referred to as a "molecular portrait" [9]. This multi-omics approach acknowledges the intricate and dynamic interplay of various molecular layers that collectively define an individual's unique health state, disease susceptibility, progression, and response to treatment. This holistic understanding allows for far more nuanced, precise, and dynamic tailoring of therapeutic interventions. This trend signifies an exponential increase in volume, velocity, and variety of heterogeneous data required for truly effective personalized medicine. It creates immense challenges for data governance, secure storage, scalable processing, and robust privacy mechanisms. Furthermore, it implies a growing and urgent need for even more sophisticated AI techniques capable of integrating and interpreting such high-dimensional, multi-modal datasets, as well as for the development of new interdisciplinary scientific expertise at the intersection of biology, advanced data science, and clinical practice. The future trajectory of personalized medicine will be profoundly shaped by our collective ability to effectively manage, integrate, and extract actionable value from this ever-growing data deluge.

5.2.5 Example of AI Applications for Genomic Profiling and Treatment Alignment

Genomic profiling involves analyzing an individual's genetic makeup to predict disease risk, prognosis, or response to treatment. AI plays a crucial role in interpreting this vast and complex data to align patients with the most effective therapies (e.g., in pharmacogenomics or oncology). The conceptual approach is as follows: (a) data integration, combine various omics data (genomics, transcriptomics, proteomics, epigenomics) with clinical data (EHRs, pathology reports); (b) biomarker discovery, AI identifies genetic variations (SNPs, mutations, gene expression patterns) that serve as biomarkers for drug response or disease susceptibility; (c) predictive modeling, train machine learning models to predict individual patient response to different drugs based on their unique genomic and clinical profiles; and (d) decision support, integrate AI models into clinical decision support systems to provide real-time treatment recommendations. An example of this approach is **Personalized Cancer Treatment Recommendation (Conceptual)**. In this example, we simulate a scenario where a machine learning model recommends a cancer treatment based on a patient's tumor genomic profile (mutations) and their response to previous treatments.

```
import pandas as pd
import numpy as np
from sklearn.model_selection import train_test_split
from sklearn.ensemble import RandomForestClassifier
from sklearn.metrics import classification_report, accuracy_score
from sklearn.preprocessing import LabelEncoder

# --- 1. Simulate a Larger, More Realistic Dataset ---
num_patients = 10000

# Let's add more complexity to the data
# We'll create rules to make the data learnable, not just random
np.random.seed(42) # for reproducibility

data = {
    'PatientID': [f'P{i:05d}' for i in range(1, num_patients + 1)],
    'Mutation_EGFR': np.random.choice([0, 1], num_patients, p=[0.8, 0.2]),
    'Mutation_KRAS': np.random.choice([0, 1], num_patients, p=[0.7, 0.3]),
    'Mutation_TP53': np.random.choice([0, 1], num_patients, p=[0.5, 0.5]),
    'Mutation_BRAF': np.random.choice([0, 1], num_patients, p=[0.9, 0.1]), # New
mutation
    'Age': np.random.randint(30, 85, size=num_patients),
    'Tumor_Stage': np.random.choice(['I', 'II', 'III', 'IV'], num_patients, p=[0.2,
0.3, 0.3, 0.2]),
    'Previous_Therapy_Response': np.random.choice(['Good', 'Poor', 'None'], num_pa-
tients, p=[0.4, 0.4, 0.2])
}
df_patients = pd.DataFrame(data)

# --- Create a "learnable" target variable based on rules ---
# This simulates how clinical decisions might be made
treatments = []
for i, row in df_patients.iterrows():
    if row['Mutation_EGFR'] == 1 and row['Tumor_Stage'] in ['I', 'II']:
        treatments.append('TreatmentA_EGFR_Targeted')
    elif row['Mutation_BRAF'] == 1:
        treatments.append('TreatmentD_BRAF_Inhibitor')
    elif row['Mutation_KRAS'] == 1 and row['Age'] > 60:
        treatments.append('TreatmentB_KRAS_Pathway')
    elif row['Tumor_Stage'] == 'IV' or row['Previous_Therapy_Response'] == 'Poor':
        treatments.append('TreatmentC_Aggressive_Chemo')
    else:
        treatments.append('Standard_Care')

df_patients['Recommended_Treatment'] = treatments

print("--- Simulated Patient Genomic and Clinical Data (First 5 of 10,000) ---")
print(df_patients.head())

# --- 2. Preprocess Data ---
# Convert categorical features to numerical using Label Encoding
# We create a dictionary of encoders to keep track of them
encoders = {}
for col in ['Tumor_Stage', 'Previous_Therapy_Response', 'Recommended_Treatment']:
    le = LabelEncoder()
    df_patients[f'{col}_Encoded'] = le.fit_transform(df_patients[col])
    encoders[col] = le # Store the encoder

# Features (X) and Target (y)
features = ['Mutation_EGFR', 'Mutation_KRAS', 'Mutation_TP53', 'Mutation_BRAF',
'Age',
            'Tumor_Stage_Encoded', 'Previous_Therapy_Response_Encoded']
X = df_patients[features]
y = df_patients['Recommended_Treatment_Encoded']

# Split data into training and testing sets (70% train, 30% test)
X_train, X_test, y_train, y_test = train_test_split(X, y, test_size=0.3, ran-
dom_state=42, stratify=y)
```

```
print("\n--- Encoded Data (Features and Target) ---")
print(X.head())
print("\nTarget Variable (Encoded):")
print(y.head())

# --- 3. Train a Machine Learning Model ---
# RandomForestClassifier is excellent for this type of complex, rule-based data
model = RandomForestClassifier(n_estimators=100, random_state=42, n_jobs=-1) # Use
all available CPU cores
model.fit(X_train, y_train)

# --- 4. Evaluate the Model ---
y_pred = model.predict(X_test)

# Retrieve the original class names for the report
target_names = encoders['Recommended_Treatment'].classes_

accuracy = accuracy_score(y_test, y_pred)
print(f"\nModel Accuracy on {len(X_test)} test patients: {accuracy:.4f}")
print("\nClassification Report:")
# Set zero_division=0 to handle cases where a class might not have any predictions
in a batch
print(classification_report(y_test, y_pred, target_names=target_names, zero_divi-
sion=0))

# --- 5. Make a Prediction for a New Patient ---
# The new patient must have all the same features the model was trained on
new_patient_data_dict = {
    'Mutation_EGFR': [1],
    'Mutation_KRAS': [0],
    'Mutation_TP53': [1],
    'Mutation_BRAF': [0],
    'Age': [58],
    # Use the stored encoders to transform the new patient's categorical data
    'Tumor_Stage_Encoded': [encoders['Tumor_Stage'].transform(['II'])[0]],
    'Previous_Therapy_Response_Encoded': [encoders['Previous_Therapy_Re-
sponse'].transform(['Good'])[0]]
}
new_patient_df = pd.DataFrame(new_patient_data_dict)


predicted_treatment_encoded = model.predict(new_patient_df)

# Use the stored treatment encoder to get the human-readable treatment name
predicted_treatment = encoders['Recommended_Treatment'].inverse_transform(pre-
dicted_treatment_encoded)

print(f"\n--- Prediction for a New Patient ---")
print(f"New Patient Profile:\n{new_patient_df.to_string(index=False)}")
print(f"\nPredicted Treatment: {predicted_treatment[0]}")
```

In this example, a large dataset of 10,000 patients is generated. Crucially, the "Recommended Treatment" is not random but is assigned based on a set of logical rules involving genetic mutations and clinical data, creating realistic and learnable patterns. Categorical text data, such as Tumor_Stage and Previous_Therapy_Response, is converted into a numerical format using LabelEncoder, making it compatible for machine learning model training. A RandomForestClassifier is trained on a 70% subset of the data. The model learns the complex, rule-based relationships between a patient's complete profile and the most effective treatment assigned during data simulation. The model's ability to generalize is rigorously tested on the remaining 30% of unseen data. Its performance is measured by its overall accuracy and a detailed classification report, which breaks down its predictive power for each treatment class. The fully trained model is used to predict a personalized treatment for a new patient. By inputting the new patient's profile, the model provides an evidence-based recommendation, demonstrating its function as a clinical decision support tool. The output of this code is as follows:

```
Classification Report:
                              precision    recall  f1-score   support

               Standard_Care       1.00      1.00      1.00       975
     TreatmentA_EGFR_Targeted       1.00      1.00      1.00       290
      TreatmentB_KRAS_Pathway       1.00      1.00      1.00       329
TreatmentC_Aggressive_Chemo       1.00      1.00      1.00      1135
   TreatmentD_BRAF_Inhibitor       1.00      1.00      1.00       271

                    accuracy                           1.00      3000
                   macro avg       1.00      1.00      1.00      3000
                weighted avg       1.00      1.00      1.00      3000


--- Prediction for a New Patient ---
New Patient Profile:
 Mutation_EGFR  Mutation_KRAS  Mutation_TP53  Mutation_BRAF  Age  Tumor_Stage_Encoded  Previous_Therapy_Response_Encoded
             1              0              1              0   58                    1                                  0

Predicted Treatment: TreatmentA_EGFR_Targeted
```

This output demonstrates a highly successful machine learning model for recommending personalized medical treatments. The classification report shows that the model achieved 100% accuracy on the 3000 test cases it was evaluated on, meaning it made no mistakes in predicting the correct treatment based on a patient's profile. The "Prediction for a New Patient" shows the model in action given a new patient with a specific set of characteristics (like having the EGFR mutation); it correctly applied the learned rules to predict the optimal treatment, which in this case was TreatmentA_EGFR_Targeted.

5.3 AI Applications in Rare and Orphan Diseases

Rare diseases, defined as conditions affecting a small percentage of the population (e.g., no more than 1 in 2000 people in the EU or fewer than 200,000 Americans in the USA), collectively impact a significant global population, estimated between 300 and 400 million people worldwide [12]. Despite this substantial collective burden, drug development for these conditions faces unique and formidable challenges.

5.3.1 Unique Challenges in Rare and Orphan Diseases

The unique challenges in rare and orphan diseases are as follows:

- **Diagnostic Odyssey:** Patients suffering from rare diseases frequently embark on a prolonged and frustrating "diagnostic odyssey," often enduring an average wait of 4–6 years to receive an accurate diagnosis [12]. This arduous journey is primarily attributable to several factors: the sheer numerical vastness of rare diseases (estimated between 6000 and 7000 distinct conditions), the remarkable diversity and variability of symptoms even within the same condition, significant symptoms overlap with more common diseases, and the tendency for rare diseases to affect multiple organ systems simultaneously [12]. This often results in a cycle of multiple misdiagnoses, ineffective or inappropriate treatments, and imposes substantial physical, emotional, and financial burdens on patients and their families [12].
- **Data Scarcity and Limited Patient Populations:** A formidable hurdle in drug development for rage diseases is the inherent limitation of patient research information and the small patient population sizes. This makes it exceedingly difficult to obtain sufficient, meaningful, and abundant datasets required for robust research, clinical trials, and statistical validation [2].
- **Heterogeneous Symptoms and Genetic Variations:** Symptoms of rare diseases can vary widely even among individuals with the same diagnosis, and many rare diseases exhibit extensive genetic variations. This heterogeneity makes consistent pattern recognition and the development of standardized treatment protocols exceptionally challenging for human clinicians [2].
- **Shortage of Specialists and Clinician Awareness:** A contributing factor to delayed diagnoses is the limited awareness of rare conditions among general clinicians and a critical shortage of specialists with expertise in these highly specific diseases [13].

5.3.2 How AI Addresses These Challenges

Artificial intelligence offers transformative solutions to these unique challenges, significantly accelerating progress in rare and orphan disease research and treatment:

- **Accelerating Diagnosis:** AI directly and significantly shortens the diagnostic odyssey by revolutionizing the diagnostic process through its ability to rapidly and accurately analyze vast amounts of medical data [12].

- **AI-Assisted Symptom Recognition and Pattern Matching:** Machine learning tools analyze extensive medical data, including patient histories, clinical notes, and research publications, to identify complex symptom patterns indicative of rare diseases. These algorithms often employ deep learning techniques and can detect subtle correlations and connections between seemingly disparate symptoms that might be missed by human clinicians, thereby enhancing diagnostic accuracy and accelerating the recognition of ultra-rare diseases [13].
- **Medical Image Analysis:** AI and machine learning can analyze medical images to detect subtle abnormalities and differentiate between positive and negative results, sometimes even beyond human capability, allowing for earlier identification of potential rare disease indicators [12].
- **Specialized AI Tools:** Examples include FindZebra, an AI powered search engine designed to aid physicians in diagnosing rare conditions by using natural language processing (NLP) to match patient symptoms with extensive medical literature [12]. The undiagnosed diseases network (UDN) utilizes AI-driven tools to compare individual patient cases with a global database of rare diseases, identifying similarities and patterns that accelerate diagnosis by connecting patients with similar cases worldwide [13].

- **Accelerating Drug Discovery:** AI directly and significantly shortens the diagnostic odyssey by revolutionizing the diagnostic process through its ability to rapidly and accurately analyze vast amounts of medical data [14].
  - AI algorithms can examine billions of chemical compounds and generate predictive drug target interaction models with exceptional precision much faster than traditional methodologies [14].
  - AI is uniquely capable of processing small datasets, which are essential for rare disease research [14]. It can combine limited genetic data with external literature and adverse event reports to highlight potential therapeutic strategies [1]. Companies like Healx and Insilico Medicine leverage AI platforms to analyze various information sources, from which new therapeutic goals can be extracted [14].
  - Atomwise and BenevolentAI utilize AI technology to enable rapid molecule searches for drugs demonstrating therapeutic promise. By analyzing extensive datasets, their algorithms generate predictions about which chemical compounds have a higher probability of success in preclinical testing, thereby lowering the possibility of experimental failure [14]. Moderna and Genentech are examples of genetic research companies that employ AI to create RNA treatments specifically targeting rare genetic conditions, producing drugs designed to eradicate essential disease origins [14].
  - Given the extensive genetic variations often observed in rare diseases, personalized medicine becomes a mandatory and highly effective approach to the treatment [14].

  - The application of AI enables highly personalized medical treatments that optimize recovery results for patients. Machine learning systems study genomic information to detect genetic fault connections with uncommon medical conditions. The combination of AI platforms with power-based algorithms design drugs that specifically target mutational variances, creating highly effective therapeutic solutions [14].
  - Al algorithms have been instrumental in identifying novel genetic mutations and suggesting targeted therapies in rage genetic disorders, leading to improved prognoses [2].
- **Clinical Trial Optimization:** AI powered platforms address the difficulties of conducting clinical trials for rage diseases, which are often characterized by small, isolated patient populations [14].
  - AI facilitates the rapid identification of qualified patients through predictive analytics systems [14]. It also advances trial designs with operational efficiency as a principal objective and enables real-time patient monitoring to minimize dropout numbers [14[. Predictive analysis through AI creates trial design improvements that boost success rates even with minimal patient involvement [14].
- **Cost-Effective Solutions:** High budget requirements traditionally deter pharmaceutical firms from investing in rare disease drug development. AI-based drug discovery tools are fundamentally changing this by automating processes for compound screening and preclinical testing, which traditionally require significant manual labor [14].
  - AI enables early detection of potential failures, preventing expensive problems in later development stages. This leads to significant cost reductions, improving the financial viability of developing medicines for rare diseases [14]. Recursion pharmaceuticals, for instance, use AI algorithms to automate cell imaging procedures and compound identification by reducing research spending [14].

5.3.3 Case Studies of Successful AI Applications

A notable case study involves the use of an AI tool to uncover a life-saving repurposed treatment for a patient with idiopathic multicentric Castleman's disease (iMCD), a rage and often fatal disease. After screening 4000 existing medications, the AI system helped identify adalimumab, a monoclonal antibody already FDA approved for conditions like arthritis and Crohn's disease, as a potential therapy. Parallel experiments confirmed that tumor necrosis factor (TNF), which adalimumab inhibits played a key role in iMCD. This led to the successful treatment of a patient who has been entering hospice care, now in remission for nearly 2 years [15]. This case powerfully illustrates the importance and efficacy of combining AI predictions with rigorous laboratory work and clinical research, rather than relying on any single approach in isolation [15].

5.3.4 Broader Implications of AI in Rare and Orphan Diseases

The integration of AI into rare disease drug development carries significant implications, particularly in transforming the economic landscape of orphan drug development. Traditionally, the high budget requirements, lengthy timelines, and notoriously low success rates associated with drug development for small patient populations have significantly deterred pharmaceutical firms from investing in these areas. AI's ability to automate complex processes, accelerate lead identification, predict potential failures early in the pipeline, and optimize clinical trial designs fundamentally alters this economic equation [14]. By substantially reducing the prohibitive R&D costs and mitigating inherent risks, AI makes the development of orphan drugs more financially viable and attractive to pharmaceutical companies. This economic shift has profound societal implications that extend beyond mere scientific advancement. If AI-driven cost-efficiencies make rare disease drug development inherently more profitable or less risky, it could lead to a significant increase in research and development efforts, ultimately resulting in a greater number of available treatments for previously neglected or underserved conditions. This transforms the issue from a purely scientific or philanthropic endeavor into a market-driven ethical imperative, where AI facilitates the delivery of therapies to patient populations that were historically overlooked due to economic disincentives. This could also influence public policy, potentially reducing the need for certain government incentives if AI makes these ventures inherently more self-sustaining.

Furthermore, while rare diseases are characterized by inherently small patient populations and thus limited individual datasets, AI's unique strength lies not just in its ability to extract patterns from these limited individual data points, but crucially, in its capacity to integrate and synthesize them with broader, often disparate, data sources [14]. This includes combining genetic data with medical records, patient registries, scientific literature, and adverse event reports. This intelligent aggregation, facilitated by AI, effectively creates larger, more comprehensive "virtual" datasets for analysis, thereby compensating for the inherent scarcity of individual patient data and enabling more robust insights. This highlights a critical aspect of AI's success in rare diseases: it is not solely about the sophistication of the algorithms, but equally about the maturity of the data infrastructure and the strength of collaborative data-sharing initiatives. The future of rare disease treatment will heavily depend on fostering robust data ecosystems that allow for the ethical and efficient pooling and analysis of diverse information, underscoring the need for inter-institutional and international cooperation to unlock the full potential of AI for these conditions.

5.3.5 Practical Example of AI in Rare and Orphan Diseases

Rare and orphan diseases pose unique challenges: small patient populations, diagnostic odysseys, scattered data, and a lack of dedicated research and drug development. AI can significantly alleviate these challenges. The conceptual approach of AI in this area is as follows:

- **Accelerated Diagnosis:** AI analyzes symptoms, medical images, genetic data, and EHRs to identify patterns indicative of rare diseases, shortening the "diagnostic odyssey."
- **Drug Discovery and Repositioning:** Overcome data scarcity by identifying subtle patterns in limited datasets, simulating molecular interactions, and predicting drug efficacy for specific rare conditions.
- **Patient Identification for Clinical Trials:** AI can sift through vast amounts of fragmented data to find eligible patients, addressing the challenge of small, dispersed patient populations.
- **Personalized Treatment:** Given the high genetic heterogeneity often seen in rare diseases, AI helps tailor treatments to individual patient's unique genetic variations.

The below code illustrates how AI might assist in diagnosing a rare disease by integrating various data points (symptoms, genetic markers). The explanation of the code is as follows:

- **Simulated Data:** Small datasets are created to represent patient symptoms, genetic markers, disease status, or drug molecular features and their effects on a disease pathway.
- **Preprocessing and Model Training:** Like the previous example, data is prepared, and a DecisionTreeClassifier is trained. Decision trees are often favored for initial exploration in rare diseases due to their interpretability.
- **Diagnostic Assistance:** The trained model takes a new patient's profile and predicts the likelihood of the rare disease, helping clinicians narrow down possibilities and shorten the "diagnostic odyssey."
- **Conceptual Drug Repositioning for Rare Diseases:** The second part demonstrates a conceptual idea where a new drug's features are compared to those of drugs known to affect a rare disease pathway. This hints at how AI, even with limited data, can identify promising candidates by finding subtle similarities or patterns. In real applications, this would involve more advanced techniques like few-shot learning, meta-learning, or sophisticated feature engineering from biological networks.

```
import pandas as pd
from sklearn.model_selection import train_test_split
from sklearn.tree import DecisionTreeClassifier
from sklearn.metrics import accuracy_score, classification_report
from sklearn.preprocessing import LabelEncoder
import numpy as np
from sklearn.metrics.pairwise import cosine_similarity
# --- 1. Simulate Data ---
# Data for patients, some with a rare disease, some without.
# 'Symptom_A' to 'Symptom_E' could be specific clinical manifestations.
# 'Genetic_Marker_X' and 'Genetic_Marker_Y' are simplified genetic predispositions.
data_rare_disease = {
    'PatientID': [f'RP{i:03d}' for i in range(1, 11)],
    'Symptom_A': [0, 1, 1, 0, 1, 0, 1, 1, 0, 1], # 1 if symptom present, 0 if not
    'Symptom_B': [1, 0, 1, 1, 0, 1, 1, 0, 1, 0],
    'Symptom_C': [0, 1, 0, 1, 1, 0, 0, 1, 0, 1],
    'Symptom_D': [1, 0, 0, 0, 1, 1, 1, 0, 1, 0],
    'Symptom_E': [0, 1, 1, 1, 0, 0, 1, 1, 0, 1],
    'Genetic_Marker_X': [1, 1, 0, 0, 1, 0, 1, 1, 0, 1],
    'Genetic_Marker_Y': [0, 0, 1, 1, 0, 1, 0, 0, 1, 0],
    'Rare_Disease_Present': ['No', 'Yes', 'No', 'Yes', 'Yes', 'No', 'Yes', 'Yes',
'No', 'Yes'] # Target variable
}
df_rare_disease = pd.DataFrame(data_rare_disease)

print("--- Simulated Rare Disease Patient Data ---")
print(df_rare_disease.head())

# --- 2. Preprocess Data ---
# Features (X) and Target (y)
features = [col for col in df_rare_disease.columns if col.startswith(('Symptom',
'Genetic_Marker'))]
X = df_rare_disease[features]

le_disease = LabelEncoder()
y = le_disease.fit_transform(df_rare_disease['Rare_Disease_Present']) # 1 for
'Yes', 0 for 'No'

# Split data into training and testing sets
X_train, X_test, y_train, y_test = train_test_split(X, y, test_size=0.3, ran-
dom_state=42) # Small dataset for demo

print("\n--- Encoded Data (Features and Target) ---")
print(X.head())
print(y[:5])

# --- 3. Train a Machine Learning Model ---
# Decision Tree Classifier, often used for its interpretability (can visualize
rules)
model = DecisionTreeClassifier(random_state=42)
model.fit(X_train, y_train)
# --- 4. Evaluate the Model ---
y_pred = model.predict(X_test)
accuracy = accuracy_score(y_test, y_pred)
print(f"\nModel Accuracy: {accuracy:.2f}")
print("\nClassification Report:")
print(classification_report(y_test, y_pred, target_names=le_disease.classes_))
# --- 5. Predict for a New Patient (Diagnostic Assistance) ---
# New patient presents with symptoms and genetic markers
new_patient_symptoms = pd.DataFrame({
    'Symptom_A': [1],
    'Symptom_B': [0],
    'Symptom_C': [1],
    'Symptom_D': [0],
    'Symptom_E': [1],
    'Genetic_Marker_X': [1],
    'Genetic_Marker_Y': [0]
})
```

```
predicted_diagnosis_encoded = model.predict(new_patient_symptoms)
predicted_diagnosis = le_disease.inverse_transform(predicted_diagnosis_encoded)

print(f"\n--- Diagnostic Prediction for a New Patient ---")
print(f"New Patient Profile:\n{new_patient_symptoms.to_string(index=False)}")
print(f"Predicted Diagnosis: {predicted_diagnosis[0]}")

# --- Example 2: Conceptual Drug Repositioning for a Rare Disease (Limited Data) --
-
# For rare diseases, often a very small dataset. AI models might need to be
# more robust to small data or use transfer learning.

# Simulate a tiny dataset for a rare disease
rare_disease_drug_data = {
    'Drug': ['RareDrug1', 'RareDrug2', 'RareDrug3'],
    'Molecular_Feature_1': [0.1, 0.9, 0.4],
    'Molecular_Feature_2': [0.8, 0.2, 0.7],
    'Effect_on_Rare_Disease_Pathway': [1, 0, 1] # 1 if positive effect, 0 if no ef-
fect
}
df_rare_drug = pd.DataFrame(rare_disease_drug_data)

# Let's say we have a new drug we want to test for repositioning
new_drug_features = np.array([[0.2, 0.6]]) # New drug has features similar to Ra-
reDrug1 and RareDrug3

# In a real scenario, this would be a more sophisticated model trained on
# complex drug-target interaction data for similar (but not identical) pathways
# or using few-shot learning techniques.
# For simplicity, we just use a similarity measure here.
print("\n--- Conceptual Drug Repositioning for a Rare Disease ---")
print("Simulated Rare Disease Drug Data:\n", df_rare_drug)

# Calculate similarity of new drug to existing drugs based on molecular features
existing_drug_features = df_rare_drug[['Molecular_Feature_1', 'Molecular_Fea-
ture_2']].values
similarities = cosine_similarity(new_drug_features, existing_drug_features)

print(f"\nSimilarities of new drug to existing drugs: {similarities[0]}")

# If similarity to a known effective drug is high, suggest it for repositioning
for i, drug in enumerate(df_rare_drug['Drug']):
    if df_rare_drug.loc[i, 'Effect_on_Rare_Disease_Pathway'] == 1 and similari-
ties[0][i] > 0.8:
        print(f"New drug is similar to '{drug}' (known to have positive effect).
Consider repositioning!")
```

The output of the code is given below. In terms of the output, the Classification Report shows a perfect accuracy of 1.00, with perfect precision, recall, and f1-scores for both yes and no cases. While this looks ideal, the support column reveals that the model was only tested on three total patients (two "no" and one "yes"). Achieving a perfect score on such a tiny test set is a classic sign of overfitting. This means the model has likely memorized the specific patterns in the small amount of data it was tested on, rather than learning general rules that would apply to new, unseen patients. As a result, the model's seemingly perfect performance is misleading and not reliable in real applications.

```
Model Accuracy: 1.00

Classification Report:
              precision    recall  f1-score   support

          No       1.00      1.00      1.00         2
         Yes       1.00      1.00      1.00         1

    accuracy                           1.00         3
   macro avg       1.00      1.00      1.00         3
weighted avg       1.00      1.00      1.00         3


--- Diagnostic Prediction for a New Patient ---
New Patient Profile:
 Symptom_A  Symptom_B  Symptom_C  Symptom_D  Symptom_E  Genetic_Marker_X  Genetic_Marker_Y
         1          0          1          0          1                 1                 0
Predicted Diagnosis: Yes

--- Conceptual Drug Repositioning for a Rare Disease ---
Simulated Rare Disease Drug Data:
        Drug  ...  Effect_on_Rare_Disease_Pathway
0  RareDrug1  ...                               1
1  RareDrug2  ...                               0
2  RareDrug3  ...                               1

[3 rows x 4 columns]

Similarities of new drug to existing drugs: [0.98058068 0.51449576 0.98058068]
New drug is similar to 'RareDrug1' (known to have positive effect). Consider repositioning!
New drug is similar to 'RareDrug3' (known to have positive effect). Consider repositioning!
```

The summary of this chapter is as follows: artificial intelligence is revolutionizing drug repurposing and personalized medicine, especially in the realm of rare diseases. Advanced machine learning models enable the discovery of new drug candidates and the tailoring of treatments to individual genetic profiles by analyzing multi-omics data. This approach accelerates accurate diagnoses, optimizes clinical trials for small patient populations, and reduces the financial risks associated with drug development, ultimately providing hope for conditions that have long lacked effective therapies.

However, as AI becomes more integrated into healthcare, it is essential to address ethical challenges, such as ensuring data privacy, preventing algorithmic bias, and promoting equitable access to AI-driven innovations. Ongoing efforts by regulatory bodies are establishing guidelines for transparency, accountability, and risk management. The responsible adoption of AI built on robust data, interdisciplinary expertise, and strong governance holds the promise of safer, more effective, and accessible treatments for all.

References

1. How is AI used for drug repurposing in biopharma? Weblink: https://synapse.patsnap.com/article/how-is-ai-used-for-drug-repurposing-in-biopharma. Accessed June 2025.
2. Nelson J. AI in personalized medicine: tailoring treatments based on patient data. 2025.
3. AI Driven Drug Discovery: 5 Powerful Breakthroughs in 2025—Lifebit. Weblink: https://lifebit.ai/blog/ai-driven-drug-discovery/. Accessed June 2025.
4. Wan Z, Sun X, Li Y, Chu T, Hao X, Cao Y, Zhang P. Applications of artificial intelligence in drug repurposing. Adv Sci. 2025;12(14):2411325.
5. Abdullahi, T., Gemou, I., Nayak, N. V., Murtaza, G., Bach, S. H., Eickhoff, C., & Singh, R. (2025). K-paths: reasoning over graph paths for drug repurposing and drug interaction prediction. arXiv preprint arXiv:2502.13344.
6. Ferreira FJ, Carneiro AS. AI-driven drug discovery: a comprehensive review. ACS Omega. 2025;10:23889.
7. FDA guidance on use of AI in drug development. Weblink: https://www.pharmalex.com/thought-leadership/blogs/how-the-fda-guidance-on-the-use-of-ai-will-impact-drug-development/. Accessed June 2025.
8. AI in pharmacogenomics: a comprehensive guide. Weblink: https://www.numberanalytics.com/blog/ai-in-pharmacogenomics-guide. Accessed June 2025.
9. Taofeek A, Oluwaferanmi A, Hamzah F, Philp A, Liang B, John B. Intergrating multi-omics data using AI in Pharamacogenomics. 2025. Weblink: https://www.researchgate.net/publication/392082901_Integrating_Multi-Omics_Data_Using_AI_in_Pharmacogenomics. Accessed June 2025.
10. What AI platforms are used for multi-omics data analysis in precision medicine? Weblink: https://synapse.patsnap.com/article/what-ai-platforms-are-used-for-multi-omics-data-analysis-in-precision-medicine. Accessed June 2025.
11. The future of pharmacogenomics: AI-powered breakthroughs. Weblink: https://www.numberanalytics.com/blog/future-of-pharmacogenomics-ai-breakthroughs. Accessed June 2025.
12. The diagnostic odyssey: The search for answers for rage diseases. Weblink: https://medicovergenetics.com/the-diagnostic-odyssey-the-search-for-answers-for-rare-diseases/. Accessed June 2025.
13. A Look At AI-Driven Medtech for Rare Disease Diagnosis. Weblink: https://www.meddeviceonline.com/doc/a-look-at-ai-driven-medtech-for-rare-disease-diagnosis-0001. Accessed June 2025.
14. How AI is addressing drug development challenges in rare diseases? Weblink: https://www.pharmafocuseurope.com/articles/how-ai-is-addressing-drug-development-challenges-in-rare-diseases. Accessed June 2025.
15. AI Drug Repurposing Helps Find Medicine for Rare Disease. Weblink: https://www.technologynetworks.com/drug-discovery/news/ai-drug-repurposing-helps-find-medicine-for-rare-disease-395863. Accessed June 2025.

Regulatory, Ethical, and Data Challenges 6

Artificial intelligence (AI) is rapidly transforming the pharmaceutical industry, offering unprecedented opportunities to accelerate drug discovery, enhance clinical trial planning, and customize treatments. By leveraging advanced AI technologies such as machine learning (ML), deep learning (DL), and natural language processing (NLP), AI systems can make more precise predictions of drug effectiveness, toxicity, and patient outcomes from extensive biological and chemical datasets [1]. This technological integration holds the potential to significantly reduce the duration and expenses associated with bringing new medications to market, a process traditionally characterized by lengthy timelines of 10–15 years and multi-billion-dollar investments, coupled with high failure rates [2].

However, alongside this transformative potential, the widespread integration of AI introduces complex regulatory, ethical, and data challenges that demand meticulous attention to ensure responsible and effective deployment. These challenges span from safeguarding sensitive patient information and navigating evolving regulatory landscapes to building trust in opaque AI models and ensuring equitable access to AI-driven innovations. This chapter will delve deeper into these critical areas, highlighting current concerns, proposed solutions, and future directions for the responsible integration of AI in drug discovery and development.

6.1 Data Privacy and Security in AI Applications

The efficacy of AI in drug discovery is profoundly dependent on access to vast quantities of high-quality, diverse data, including sensitive genomic information and electronic health records (EHRs). This reliance, however, introduces significant privacy and security challenges that necessitate robust frameworks and continuous vigilance.

K. Shaikh et al., *Artificial Intelligence in Drug Discovery and Development*,
Synthesis Lectures on Engineering, Science, and Technology,
https://doi.org/10.1007/978-3-032-10277-5_6

6.1.1 Core Privacy Concerns and Re-identification Risks

The collection, use, analysis, and sharing of health data for AI applications raise substantial concerns regarding individual privacy [3]. The potential harms extend beyond mere data breaches to include future discrimination based on health status, a loss of dignity if sensitive data is improperly shared, and a broader erosion of public trust in healthcare systems and research institutions [4]. Even AI-generated recommendations can themselves raise privacy concerns, as individuals may expect these "new" health data to remain private [3]. These concerns are particularly heightened for stigmatized and vulnerable populations, where data disclosure could lead to discrimination or punitive measures [4].

A significant ethical and legal concern is the phenomenon known as "behavioral data surplus" or "function creep." This occurs when health data initially collected by technology providers for a specific purpose exceeds what is required and is subsequently repurposed for other uses, such as sharing with government agencies for control or punitive measures, often without explicit consent [3]. The commercialization of health data further compounds this issue, potentially leading to an individual's loss of autonomy and control over their own information, with companies potentially profiting from data without explicit consent for secondary use [3].

Traditional privacy safeguards, such as informed consent, duty of confidentiality, and deidentification, are frequently insufficient in the context of AI and biomedical big data [3]. Deidentification techniques, while aiming to remove identifiable information, are not foolproof [5]. Sophisticated "data triangulation" techniques can reidentify individual from incomplete datasets, and some data, such as genome sequences, may be inherently impossible to fully deidentify [4]. It may be inherently impossible to fully deidentify [5]. Furthermore, masked data may not accurately reflect real-world scenarios or may remain vulnerable to re-identification, and data generalization, while protecting privacy, can decrease granularity, leading to the loss of important distinctions critical for AI analysis [6]. The increasing reliance on vast, heterogeneous datasets, including genomic data and EHRs, for AI training directly amplifies the risk of re-identification, even when advanced anonymization techniques are employed. This is because AI's sophisticated analytical capabilities can infer patterns and link seemingly disparate data points, thereby rendering traditional deidentification less robust over time.

While the concern about reidentification of genomic data through linkage with public face images is a valid consideration, recent research suggests that the practical risk might be lower than some initial claims, particularly in larger populations. Studies indicate that the actual risk posed by linkage attacks to typical face images is substantially smaller than suggested in prior investigations [7]. Moreover, this risk can be mitigated with the addition of "imperceptible noise" to images, which can markedly reduce the reidentification success rate [7]. This observation underscores the need for a nuanced risk assessment rather than blanket assumptions, allowing for more proportionate and effective privacy strategies. The commercialization and repurpose of health data, enabled by AI's powerful processing capabilities, threaten individual autonomy and possess the potential to exacerbate health inequities by creating new forms of discrimination, thereby undermining the ethical foundation of AI in healthcare.

6.1.2 Evolving Cybersecurity Threats to AI in Pharma R&D

The increasing reliance on AI-driven processes in pharmaceutical research and development (R&D) exposes the industry to a new generation of sophisticated cybersecurity threats [8]. Traditional security measures are often inadequate against these evolving challenges, necessitating a fundamental shift in defensive strategies [8]. Key threats included [8]:

- **Adversarial AI Manipulations:** This broad category encompasses techniques such as model poisoning, where malicious data is injected into training sets to subtly alter how an AI model behaves. Such manipulation could lead to faulty molecular structures, incorrect biomarker identification, or misclassified drug candidates, directly endangering public health [8]. Other forms of adversarial manipulation include model fine-tuning attacks and label poisoning, where deliberately mislabeled data causes predictable errors [9].
- **Ransomware Attacks:** These attacks can specifically target and encrypt sensitive research data and AI models, causing severe disruptions to critical drug discovery pipelines and potentially halting vital research [8].
- **Data Memorization:** Healthcare AI models, particularly those trained on extensive patient records, can inadvertently memorize sensitive protected health information (PHI). This creates a risk where carefully crafted prompts from malicious actors could extract sensitive details like patient names, diagnoses, or treatment plans, even from models that appear to be properly sanitized [9].
- **Adversarial Attacks (Evasion):** AI models can be tricked with specially crafted inputs, leading them to make incorrect predictions or even reveal sensitive data. Attackers can systematically query AI systems to reconstruct sensitive patient information from the model's responses or manipulate data entries just enough to fool the model into misclassifying a disease [9].
- **Data Exfiltration:** Even when direct access to training data is restricted, AI models can inadvertently leak patient information through their APIs. Attackers can systematically query these interfaces to piece together protected health information [9].
- **Malicious Use of AI:** Cybercriminals are increasingly leveraging AI to create more sophisticated and scalable attacks. Examples include AI-generated phishing emails that mimic healthcare provider communication styles, automated vulnerability scanning of healthcare networks, deepfake voice and video tools used to impersonate authorized personnel, and automated patient data extraction from compromised systems [9]. These AI-enhanced attacks are particularly effective due to their ability to adapt to defensive measures and operate at scale.

The unique vulnerabilities inherent to AI models, such as susceptibility to data poisoning, adversarial attacks, and data memorization, mean that traditional cybersecurity approaches are insufficient. This necessitates a paradigm shift toward AI-specific security frameworks, integrating "secure-by-design" principles at every stage of AI development [10]. The direct consequence of these new threats extends beyond mere data loss, potentially leading to compromised drug integrity and direct risks to patient safety. The rapid evolution of AI capabilities for malicious use creates an "AI arms race" in cybersecurity, where defensive measures must constantly adapt to new offensive tactics. This dynamic environment demands continuous investment and innovation in AI-driven security solutions to develop resilient and adaptive security models capable of detecting and mitigating malicious activities in real time [8].

6.1.3 Current Safeguards and Their Limitations

Despite existing data protection standards, such as the general data protection regulation (GDPR) and health insurance portability and accountability act (HIPAA), significant limitations persist in safeguarding sensitive health data within AI applications. A primary concern is the anxiety stemming from the perceived lack of formal, comprehensive regulation specifically for AI in precision medicine, leading to uncertainty about who has access and control over personal health information [11]. Current mechanisms for date protection, including informed consent, confidentiality, and deidentification, are often insufficient in the face of AI's capabilities [3]. While explicit informed consent is crucial for data access, ensuring its continuous relevance and application for the vast, evolving datasets needed to train AI algorithms present an ongoing challenge [11]. Furthermore, the past decade has witnessed numerous controversies where companies allegedly exploited patient information for their gain, with data sharing occurring between companies and global health entities utilizing millions of patient health data for AI development [11]. The perceived "relaxed nature of the regulatory bodies" in monitoring and rectifying these violations exacerbates concerns among the public and industry stakeholders [11].

A notable "loophole" identified is the third-party access to deidentified patient information by researchers without explicit patient consent [11]. While deidentification aims to protect privacy, its effectiveness is limited. Advanced AI and machine learning algorithms are increasingly capable of reidentifying anonymized data, especially when combined with other demographic or publicly available information [11]. This "data triangulation" undermines the confidentiality patients expect when providing their data for research or clinical purposes [3]. Other limitations of current data anonymization techniques include:

- **Limited Effectiveness:** Some techniques may not be effective, particularly when combined with other AI-driven security measures, as the synergistic power of AI can bypass individual safeguards [5].

- **Complexity and Cost:** Implementing robust anonymization can be complex and costly, requiring significant resources and specialized technical expertise, which can act as a barrier for widespread adoption, especially for smaller entities [5].
- **Scalability Issues:** Maintaining effective anonymization across large, dynamic datasets is challenging, as the complexity of protection measures increases exponentially with data volume and change [5].
- **Lack of Standardization:** The absence of standardized anonymization techniques can lead to inconsistencies and inefficiencies in data protection across different organizations and jurisdictions [5].
- **Data Quality Degradation:** Over-anonymizing data can strip away essential details, correlations, and attributes, making the data less useful for precise decision-making or insights, particularly for critical medical research and machine learning training where roughness is key [6].

6.1.4 Advancing Data Protection: Solutions and Best Practices

Addressing the complex data privacy and security challenges in AI drug discovery requires a multifaceted approach, integrating robust technical solutions with strong governance and ethical frameworks. Key solutions and best practices include:

- **Robust Data Privacy and Security Measures:** Implementing strong encryption protocols, rigorous access controls, and secure computing environments are paramount to protect patient data from unauthorized access throughout its lifecycle [4].
- **Ethical Frameworks and Data Governance:** Establishing clear ethical frameworks that address data ownership, explicit consent, and transparent data sharing agreements is critical for building a trustworthy data ecosystem [4]. Robust data governance policies are essential for ensuring data quality, security, and compliance with evolving regulatory requirements [12].
- **AI-Driven Security Solutions:** Given the evolving nature of cyber threats, AI-driven security solutions are becoming paramount to detect and mitigate malicious activities in real time. This includes embedding "secure-by-design" principles at every stage of AI development, ensuring security is not an afterthought but an integral component [8].
- **Privacy-Preserving AI (PPAI) Techniques:** These advanced cryptographic and computational methods enable data utilization without compromising privacy, directly addressing the core tension between data utility and individual privacy:
  - **Federated Learning:** This collaborative model training method allows AI models to be trained on decentralized devices (e.g., at individual hospitals or research centers) using local data, without the data ever leaving its sources. This innovative approach preserves individual data privacy while contributing to a global model, addressing ethical concerns related to data privacy and the risks associated with centralized data storage [13].

  - **Differential Privacy:** This technique adds carefully calibrated noise to datasets or algorithm outputs, ensuring that the model does not overfit sensitive individual data. It provides a mathematical guarantee that the presence or absence of any single individual's data in the training set does not significantly alter the model's output, thereby protecting privacy while allowing for robust statistical analysis [13].
  - **Homomorphic Encryption (FHE):** This quantum-resilient cryptography method allows computations to be performed directly on encrypted data without the need for decryption. This capability enables secure analysis of patient data for advanced research and facilitates secure collaboration across multiple institutions, even in untrusted environments. FHE can bridge the gaps left by traditional encryption, which only protects data in transit and rest, by safeguarding data in use. It holds transformative potential for leveraging multi-institutional datasets for AI tools, despite current challenges related to its computational intensity and the requirement for specialized expertise [14].
- **International Collaboration and Harmonization:** Fostering international collaboration and harmonization of data privacy regulations is vital for consistent protection of patient data across borders in global AI-driven discovery initiatives. This ensures a unified approach to data governance in an increasingly interconnected research landscape [3].

Privacy-preserving AI techniques like federated learning, differential privacy, and homomorphic encryption represent a fundamental shift towards enabling data utilization without compromising privacy. Their adoption is crucial for scaling AI in drug discovery while simultaneously building and maintaining public trust. By fundamentally changing how data is processed and shared, these technologies can overcome the limitations of traditional safeguards, thereby fostering the trust necessary for large-scale data aggregation and enabling wider, more ethical adoption of AI in drug discovery. The successful implementation of these advanced data protection measures requires not only technological adoption but also robust data governance frameworks, international regulatory harmonization, and increased public literacy about AI's data handling practices. This multifaced approach, encompassing legal, ethical, and educational components, is necessary to create a truly secure and trusted data ecosystem for AI in drug discovery at a global scale.

6.2 Regulatory Frameworks for AI-Driven Tools

The rapid integration of AI across the drug development lifecycle has prompted regulatory authorities worldwide to evaluate and adapt existing frameworks to accommodate these novel technologies. This section explores the approaches taken by key regulatory bodies, the challenges they face, and future directions for AI governance in pharmaceuticals.

6.2.1 Overview of Key Regulatory Bodies and Their Approaches

Two prominent regulatory bodies, the US Food and Drug Administration (FDA) and the European Medicines Agency (EMA), have been at the forefront of developing guidance for AI in medicinal product development. Their approaches, while sharing common objectives, also exhibit distinct characteristics reflecting their respective legal and operational contexts.

The US Food and Drug Administration (FDA) released draft guidance in January 2025 titled "Considerations for the Use of Artificial Intelligence to Support Regulatory Decision-Making for Drug and Biological Products" [14, 15]. This guidance primarily focuses on AI models that directly impact patient safety, drug quality, or the reliability of results from non-clinical or clinical studies [16]. Notably, it explicitly states that AI models used solely for drug discovery or operational efficiencies that do not directly influence patient safety or product quality are generally outside its immediate scope [16]. The FDA's framework was informed by extensive stakeholder feedback, including expert workshops, over 800 public comments, and the center for drug evaluation and research's (CDER) experience with more than 500 AI-related submissions between 2016 and 2023 [17]. The agency aims to align regulatory approaches across its various medical product centers to foster a consistent and trustworthy use of AI [17].

The European Medicines Agency (EMA) published its "Reflection paper on the use of Artificial Intelligence (AI) in the medicinal product lifecycle" in September 2024 [18]. This paper adopts a broader scope, covering AI applications across the entire medicinal product lifecycle, including drug discovery, non-clinical development, clinical trials, precision medicine, product information, and post-authorization activities [18]. The EMA's approach emphasizes minimizing the integration of bias into AI/ML applications and promoting overall trustworthiness, advocating for a human-centric approach to AI development and deployment [18]. In May 2025, the EMA, in conjunction with the Heads of Medicines Agencies (HMA), launched a joint workplan "Data and AI in medicines regulation to 2028." This 5-year roadmap details how regulators will manage, analyze, and share regulatory and health data to support faster, evidence-based decision-making across the EU regulatory network, ensuring alignment with broader EU legislative initiatives such as the European Health Data Space (EHDS), the AI Act, and GDPR [19]. The European Federation of Pharmaceutical Industries and Associations (EFPIA) supports leveraging existing EU regulations and EMA oversight, arguing that AI systems used solely for medicines R&D should be exempt from the requirements of the EU AI Act to foster innovation [20].

Both the FDA and EMA are converging on a risk-based, lifecycle approach to AI regulation in drug development, reflecting a shared understanding of AI's dynamic nature and the need for adaptive oversight. However, differences in scope, particularly the FDA's initial exclusion of pure discovery AI, and the specific legal framework such as the EU AI Act, create potential for divergence in global regulatory expectations. The increasing number of AI components in drug application submissions is a primary driver for regulatory bodies to rapidly develop guidance, indicating a reactive rather than purely proactive stance to technological advancement. This continuous influx of AI-enabled products necessitates ongoing adaptation of regulatory frameworks.

6.2.2 Risk-Based Frameworks and Context of Use (COU)

Central to both FDA and EMA guidance is the adoption of a risk-based framework, with the "context of use" (COU) serving as a critical determinant for regulatory scrutiny. The FDA's guidance, for instance, proposes that the risk level posed by an AI model dictates the extent and depth of information that must be disclosed about it [16]. This risk is determined by two primary factors: "model influence risk," which assesses how much the AI model will influence decision-making, and "decision consequence risk," which evaluates the potential consequences of that decision, such as patient safety risks [16].

The FDA has outlined a seven-step credibility assessment process for AI models: (1) defining the question of interest, (2) defining the specific COU for the AI model, (3) assessing the AI model risk, (4) developing a plan to establish the credibility of the AI model output within the COU, (5) executing that plan, (6) documenting the results and discussing deviations, and (7) determining the adequacy of the AI model for its intended COU [15]. This framework emphasizes thorough validation and documentation to reduce bias and increase transparency [21]. Sponsors are required to describe the AI model, the data used for its development and training, and the model's evaluation, including test data, performance metrices and reliability concerns such as bias, quality assurance, and code error management [16]. Transparency regarding the source data used to train the AI algorithm is also expected [14], with data needing to be "fit for use," meaning relevant and reliable data for the specific COU [22]. A life cycle maintenance plan is also required to monitor and ensure the model's performance over time [16]. The level of human control over AI outputs may also vary depending on the COU [14].

The risk-based COU framework directly links regulatory scrutiny to the potential impact on patient safety and drug quality. This approach incentivizes developers to clearly define AI's role and the degree of human oversight, but it also places a significant burden on sponsors to provide extensive documentation and demonstrate data "fitness for use" and model credibility. This necessitates substantial investment in data governance, quality assurance, and detailed documentation from the outset, moving beyond mere algorithmic performance to demonstrating comprehensive regulatory readiness. The FDA's encouragement of early engagement between sponsors and the agency signals a shift toward a more collaborative regulatory process [14]. This collaborative stance highlights the inherent complexity and uncertainty that sponsors face in navigating novel AI applications without clear precedents, creating an opportunity for regulatory science to evolve dynamically alongside technological innovation.

6.2.3 Challenges in Regulating Adaptive and Evolving AI Models

One of the most profound challenges in regulating AI-driven tools stems from the inherent "adaptive" nature of advanced AI models. These models, particularly those employing continuous learning, can evolve over time or across deployment environments due to "data drift" or deliberate updates [16]. This continuous evolution introduces unique risks and biases that may not have been present or fully anticipated during pre-market evaluations [23].

The core regulatory dilemma lies in the fundamental clash between the dynamic nature of AI and traditional "locked" regulatory approval paradigms. Conventional validation approaches, designed for static medical products, are often inadequate for adaptive algorithms [23]. Consequently, regulatory authorities often advocate for "locked" models at the time of validation, requiring a predetermined change control plan (PCCP) for any subsequent updates [14]. Continuous learning models are viewed with skepticism unless robust mechanisms for tracking and auditing modifications are in place [24]. For instance, the FDA requested Moderna to "lock" its AI algorithm before a study for personalized vaccines to prevent bias from an evolving algorithm [14].

The challenge extends beyond individual models to the regulatory agencies themselves. When a proprietary AI algorithm becomes a critical component of a drug product, such as determining the mRNA sequence in personalized vaccines, it poses new challenges for traditional manufacturing inspections, which are not designed to scrutinize algorithms [14]. The FDA, for example, faces significant hurdles in rapidly acquiring the necessary resources and expertise to scrutinize these proprietary AI algorithms effectively [14]. Furthermore, there have been identified inconsistencies in how the FDA categorizes and approves these technologies [23], alongside persistent weaknesses in real-time monitoring, transparency, and bias mitigation in the post-market phase [23]. The lack of continuous large-scale prospective evaluations of AI algorithms in diverse clinical settings can lead to unintended consequences, potentially risking patient livelihood [23].

6.2.4 Future Regulatory Directions and International Harmonization

The regulatory landscape for AI in drug development is still in its nascent stages, with much of the current guidance, such as the FDA's being in draft and non-binding form, signaling an ongoing evolution [16]. The FDA anticipates releasing more specific guidance for complex contexts of use in the future [14].

Regulatory bodies are increasingly moving beyond reactive responses to AI by developing multi-year workplans and engaging stakeholders early, aiming for a more proactive and harmonized approach to AI governance. The EMA's "Data and AI in medicines regulation to 2028" workplan exemplifies this strategic shift, detailing how data and AI will be leveraged to support faster, evidence-based decision-making while ensuring alignment with broader EU legislative initiatives like the European Health Data Space (EHDS), the

AI Act, and GDPR [19]. Key milestones within this plan include the publication of responsible AI principles and a terminology guide in 2025, the establishment of an AI industry working group, and the initiation of 6-month experimentation cycles to test AI methods starting in 2026, with outcomes reviewed in 2027 [25]. The EMA aims to integrate AI across the medicines lifecycle to improve regulatory efficiency and decision-making, ensuring ethical and compliant use under EU rules [25].

Industry groups like EFPIA call for globally consistent, risk-based AI regulations. The FDA encourages early discussions with sponsors to address AI model development, fostering collaboration amid regulatory uncertainty. Both industry and regulators are adapting to draft guidance and practical experience. The success of AI in drug development depends on modernized regulations, international harmonization, and collaboration, balancing safety with innovation. While the FDA is exploring generative AI for reviewing submissions, standard practices for AI are still evolving, and challenges in risk mitigation remain.

6.3 Explainability and Trust in AI Models

The increasing reliance on AI in critical domains like drug discovery and development necessitates a profound understanding of how these complex systems arrive at their conclusions. This imperative gives rise to challenges related to explainability and, consequently, the establishment of trust among all stakeholders.

6.3.1 The "Black Box" Problem and Its Implications in Drug Discovery

Many advanced AI models, particularly those based on deep learning, operate as "black boxes" due to their complex, non-transparent model architectures [18]. This inherent opacity makes it difficult to interpret and understand by human users, including medical professionals, patients, and regulators [26]. The lack of transparency is profoundly problematic for ensuring the safety, efficacy, and fairness of AI-driven processes, especially when they involve life-and-death decisions in drug development [27].

This opaqueness directly impedes human oversight, auditability, and the ability to identify and mitigate biases, which in turn undermines regulatory acceptance and public trust. When an AI model's reasoning is obscured, it becomes challenging for evaluators to identify errors, assess the fitness of data, and ensure the reliability of its outputs [23]. This can hinder regulatory approval processes. Furthermore, deploying AI tools that lack transparency or explainability has the potential to exacerbate existing health disparities, particularly if their internal workings lead to biased outcomes for certain demographic groups [23]. Regulators increasingly expect manufacturers to understand and justify the logic behind AI predictions, moving beyond mere performance metrices to a deeper comprehension of the model's decision-making [28]. Beyond technical and regulatory compliance, the "black box" problem raises fundamental ethical questions about accountability in

AI-driven healthcare, particularly when patient lives are at stake. If a model makes a decision that leads to an adverse outcome, and its reasoning cannot be traced or understood, assigning responsibility becomes a complex ethical dilemma.

6.3.2 Importance of Explainability for Clinical Adoption and Regulatory Acceptance

Explainability and transparency are not merely regulatory checkboxes but foundational elements for building and maintaining trust among clinicians, patients, and regulators, which is essential for the widespread and ethical adoption of AI in drug discovery and clinical practice. Trust is unequivocally identified as key to facilitating the adoption of AI in medicine [3]. For AI to have a beneficial impact on public health and medicine, ethical considerations and human rights must be placed at the center of its design, development, and deployment [3].

Transparency is crucial for system evaluators to identify errors and for government regulators to conduct proper oversight [3]. It enables users to understand the benefits, risks, and limitations of AI tools [23]. Transparency also directly promotes trust among all stakeholders, particularly patients [3]. Physicians, as intermediaries, are encouraged to be candid with patients about AI used, explaining its purpose, function, data collection, sharing practices, and safeguards for privacy. This transparency should also extend to acknowledging any weaknesses, biases, data breaches, or privacy concerns [3]. Regulatory bodies are increasingly recognizing this imperative, for instance, the EU AI Act is poised to make transparency a core requirement for high-risk AI systems [29], and explainable AI (XAI) systems are expected to provide clear and understandable descriptions and explanations for user comprehension [30]. The absence of widespread trust due to opaque AI could create significant divisions in healthcare systems, potentially leading to unequal access or even outright refusal of AI-driven care, especially among older patients or those from vulnerable populations [3]. Such a scenario could exacerbate existing health disparities, leading to a two-tiered healthcare system where some benefit from AI advancements, while others are left behind due to a lack of confidence.

6.3.3 Strategies for Enhancing Explainability (XAI)

Addressing the "black box" problem requires a multi-pronged approach, collectively known as explainable AI (XAI), which focuses on creating AI models that can provide understandable explanations for their decisions [26]. Designing AI models with explainable capabilities is a critical step in this direction [16]. Key techniques and approaches for XAI include:

- **Model-Agnostic Approaches:** Techniques such as LIME (Local Interpretable Model-Agnostic Explanations) and SHAP (Shapley Additive exPlanations) can explain the predictions of any classifier by approximating its behavior locally or by assigning importance values to features for a particular prediction [28]. These methods provide understandable explanations for individual predictions, making it easier for users to comprehend the model's output [26].
- **Intrinsically Interpretable Models:** Some AI models, like decision trees and rule-based systems, are designed to be interpretable from the ground up, offering inherent transparency [26].
- **Hybrid Models:** Combining intrinsically interpretable models with high accuracy, but less transparent, models can enhance both transparency and performance, attempting to bridge the gap between interpretability and accuracy [26].
- **Explainability by Design:** This methodology advocates for building interpretable models from the ground up, rather than attempting to explain black-box models after they have been developed [28].
- **Feature Attribution Methods:** Beyond SHAP, other methods identify the most important factors contributing to a particular prediction [31].
- **Model Visualization:** Techniques such as activation maps, saliency maps, and latent space projections can provide visual insights into a model's internal workings [31].
- **Rule-Based and Symbolic Methods:** Incorporating explicit rules into AI systems can make their decision-making processes more transparent and understandable [31].
- **Counterfactual and Sensitivity Analysis:** These methods probe how variations in input affect output, helping to understand a model's robustness and dependencies [31].

A significant technical dilemma in drug discovery is the pursuit of explainability, which often involves a trade-off with model accuracy, particularly for complex deep learning models [26]. While high accuracy is paramount for safety and efficacy in drug development, explainability is crucial for regulatory approval and building trust. Effective XAI implementation requires not just technical solutions but also a holistic approach encompassing data quality, bias mitigation, and human-AI collaboration throughout the design and development lifecycle. This includes ensuring diverse and representative training data, actively spotting and mitigating biases using fairness metrics, and incorporating inclusive design processes that involve diverse stakeholders, including domain experts, affected communities, and ethicists [30].

6.3.4 Building Trust Through Transparency and Ethical Design

True trust in AI in drug discovery cannot be achieved through technical transparency alone; it requires a robust ethical governance framework that prioritizes human rights, fairness, accountability, and continuous public engagement throughout the AI lifecycle. Transparency is crucial for the long-term success and widespread adoption of AI in healthcare [3]. This necessitates sufficient information to be published or documented both before the design or deployment of AI technology and regularly after its approval, to facilitate meaningful public consultation and debate and to improve system quality and protect patient and public health safety [3]. This information should include accurate details about the technology's assumptions, limitations, operating protocols, data properties (collection, processing, labeling), and algorithmic model development.

The auditability of AI technology is also a necessary component of transparency, particularly when something goes wrong [3]. Governments are increasingly required to disclose the use of algorithms in services and operations to promote accountability and transparency [3]. Physicians play a vital role in building trust by being frank with patients about AI use, explaining its purpose, function, data collection, sharing practices, and safeguards for privacy. This transparency should also extend to openly discussing any weaknesses, biases, data breaches, or privacy concerns associated with the AI system [3].

At a foundational level, ethical considerations and human rights must be placed at the center of AI's design, development, and deployment [3]. This involves ensuring that AI systems are auditable and traceable, with robust oversight, impact assessment, audit, and due diligence mechanisms in place to avoid conflicts with human rights norms and threats to well-being [21]. Principles of fairness and non-discrimination are paramount, ensuring that AI's benefits are accessible to all [21]. A "human-centric approach" should guide all AI development and deployment, emphasizing that AI systems do not displace ultimate human responsibility and accountability [18]. Transparency should be viewed as a comprehensive system of accountability, distributed across AI developers, healthcare professionals, and patients [32]. Scandals or abuses of trust emerging from AI use could be fatal to public trust in healthcare [3], underscoring the critical need for proactive, honest communication, and robust safeguards to prevent such incidents. The willingness of patients to rely on AI may sometimes be much lower than expected, making proactive trust-building measures essential [3].

6.4 Industry-Academic Collaborations and Standardization

The complexity and capital intensity of AI-driven drug discovery necessitate a collaborative ecosystem, particularly strong partnerships between industry and academia. Concurrently, the proliferation of diverse data types and AI models underscores the critical need for standardization to ensure interoperability and data quality.

6.4.1 Benefits and Successful Models of Collaboration

Industry-academic collaborations are not merely additive but create a synergistic effect, combining academic foundational research and diverse datasets with industry's scaling capabilities and clinical translation expertise, significantly accelerating the traditionally slow and expensive drug discovery process. These partnerships are instrumental in accelerating research and development (R&D), improving efficiency, accuracy, and speed across the pharmaceutical value chain [33]. By leveraging existing safety data and pharmacological information, AI-supported drug repurposing, often a product of such collaborations, can significantly decrease development timelines from traditional 10–15 years to potentially 3–6 years, and cut costs by up to 70% through better compound selection [2]. This ultimately leads to improved patient outcomes and more customized treatments [33].

Collaborations foster the sharing of expertise and resources, establishing robust collaborative networks across academia, healthcare institutions, and regulatory bodies [32]. Access to diverse datasets, often housed within academic institutions or collected through clinical research, is a key benefit [4]. Evidence suggests the prevalence of such partnerships, with industry collaborations reported in 97% of relevant studies [34]. Notable examples of successful models, some predating widespread AI adoption but illustrating enduring principles of collaboration, include:

- AstraZeneca's partnership with AI companies like BenevolentAI and Quar.ai which have advanced treatments for kidney disease and pulmonary fibrosis faster than traditional in-house R&D [35].
- Pfizer's collaboration with IBM Watson to accelerate oncology therapies through AI's cognitive computing capabilities [36].
- DeepMind's AlphaFold, which made a groundbreaking advance in protein folding prediction, significantly aiding drug target identification and design [36].

These cases demonstrate that the principles of effective industry academic partnership are transferable and foundational with AI acting as an accelerant rather than a completely new paradigm for collaboration itself.

6.4.2 Challenges in Fostering Effective Partnerships

Despite the clear benefits, fostering effective industry-academic partnerships in AI drug discovery is fraught with challenges. Fundamentally, differing timelines between academia, driven by research cycles and publication pressures, and industry, focused on rapid commercialization and market demands, can clash [35]. Divergent incentive structures further complicate alignment [35].

Intellectual property (IP) considerations represent a significant hurdle. While IP protection is crucial for incentivizing innovation, the differing IP strategies between academia (often emphasizing open publication) and industry (prioritizing trade secrets and patents) can create substantial friction, especially when AI models themselves become proprietary "components" of drug products [16]. For instance, trade secret protection may be an option for AI models not directly impacting patient safety or drug quality, but this can conflict with transparency requirements for regulatory approval [16]. This tension between transparency, necessary for validation and trust, and trade secrets, vital for competitive advantage, is a key challenge.

Beyond IP, fundamental differences in organizational culture, operational pace, and data governance post structural barriers to seamless collaboration. Internal legacy systems, data silos, and organizational inertia within large pharmaceutical companies can significantly slow the adoption and integration of AI innovations for external partners [15]. There is also a recognized need for greater interdisciplinary collaboration, bridging the gaps between AI experts, biologists, chemists, and clinicians [37]. Furthermore, the concentration of data, computing power, and human resources within a few large technology companies can lead to monopoly power, potentially impacting equitable access to AI innovations [3]. Regulatory hurdles also remain a challenge for such partnerships [32], with some industry bodies, like EFPIA, advocating for AI systems used in R&D to be exempt from the EU AI Act's stringent requirements to avoid stifling innovation [20]. These deep-seated organizational issues require more than just legal agreements; they demand cultural shifts and robust data governance frameworks to enable effective data sharing and interoperability.

6.4.3 Role of Standardization in Interoperability and Data Quality

Standardization of data formats and robust data governance, including principles of data integrity and lineage, are not merely technical conveniences but fundamental prerequisites for building trustworthy and generalizable AI models in drug discovery. These factors directly impact regulatory approval and clinical utility. The FDA, for instance, requires that data used to train AI models be "fit for use," meaning it must be relevant and reliable for its intended purpose [16]. Thorough validation and documentation are also essential to reduce bias and ensure data quality [38]. Transparency about data properties, including collection, processing, and labeling, is crucial [3].

Data integrity is paramount, adhering to principles such as ALCOA+ (attributable, legible, contemporaneous, original, accurate, complete, consistent, enduring, available), throughout the data pipeline, from training to deployment [28]. The "digital thread" concept, referring to an unbroken chain of data relationships from raw material testing to final product release, is gaining prominence to ensure data lineage and auditability [28]. The absence of standardized data formats and vocabulary can lead to data inconsistencies and make it difficult to integrate data from different sources [12]. Regulations play a vital role in establishing common guidelines and standards for AI applications in healthcare, promoting interoperability and compatibility among different systems, which is essential for seamless collaboration and communication within the healthcare ecosystem [39].

Initiatives like HL7 FHIR (Health Level 7 Fast Healthcare Interoperability Resources) are critical for bridging the gap between real-world clinical data (EHRs) and are structured research data. FHIR serves as a standard for exchanging healthcare information electronically, providing an API for data exchange between diverse EHR applications [40]. It offers capabilities for traceability, validation, error reporting, data segmentation, and workflow integration, facilitating the pre-population of clinical research eCRFs from EHR data (eSource) [40]. Similarly, CDISC (Clinical Data Interchange Standards Consortium) is a standards development organization that has developed data standards used across the biopharmaceutical industry to harmonize clinical trial data (e.g., CDASH, SDTM, ADaM), ensuring traceability from planning to statistical analysis [24]. The EMA's workplan also emphasizes "high standards in data quality, sharing, and analytics" and "data interoperability" across the European medicine's regulatory network [25]. These efforts are vital for enabling the robust, diverse datasets necessary for advanced AI training and validation.

6.4.4 Initiatives and Future Directions for Collaborative Ecosystems

The future of AI in drug discovery relies on fostering a comprehensive, multi-stakeholder ecosystem that includes not only industry and academia but also regulatory bodies, patient groups, and technology providers, all working collaboratively to address technical, ethical, and societal challenges. This ecosystem approach is crucial for navigating the complexities of AI integration. Key initiatives and future directions include:

- **Formation of Consortiums and Innovation Centers:** Dedicated entities focused on AI integration within life sciences, health economics, and healthcare can serve as incubators for new ideas and pilot projects, fostering a shared environment for innovation [32].
- **Public-Private Partnerships:** These collaborations can align research priorities with global health needs, equitably share data and resources, and make AI innovations available to all who need it, particularly in low- and middle-income countries [4].
- **Regulatory Engagement Platforms:** The EMA's AI industry working group (established in 2025) and its digital academy, which is expanding with AI masterclasses, exemplify efforts to build capacity and facilitate dialogue [25]. The EMA's network AI observatory, designed for annual trend reports and stakeholder events like hackathons, further promotes engagement and shared learning [25].
- **Cross-Sector Working Groups:** Organizations like HL7 are actively calling on healthcare stakeholders to engage in cross-sector working groups and participate in pilots that demonstrate how AI applications, powered by interoperable data standards, can deliver faster and more accurate outcomes [40].
- **Multidisciplinary Teams:** The integration of clinical, technical, and regulatory expertise within multidisciplinary teams is vital for developing solutions that are both scientifically sound and practically implementation. External partnerships can significantly accelerate internal innovation by bringing diverse perspective and resources.
- **Ethical Imperative of Equitable Access:** Collaborative efforts must explicitly prioritize equitable access and address health disparities [4]. This ensures that the benefits of AI-driven drug discovery reach underserved populations and contribute to global health

equity, rather than exacerbating existing divides. Governments have a duty to ensure equitable access to AI-based healthcare for all, regardless of gender, geography, or ethnicity [3]. AI's potential to shorten the "diagnostic odyssey" for rate diseases, which disproportionately affects vulnerable populations, highlights its role in addressing existing inequalities. This means collaborations need to have a social justice lens, ensuring that the innovations are not just effective but also universally accessible and beneficial.

Artificial intelligence is reshaping the landscape of drug discovery, accelerating development and enhancing efficiency across the pharmaceutical sector. However, this transformation introduces significant challenges related to data privacy, security, and regulatory compliance. The reliance on extensive, high-quality, and diverse datasets for training AI systems heightens concerns around privacy and increases exposure to sophisticated cyber threats.

Regulatory bodies such as the FDA and EMA are actively updating their oversight frameworks to address the evolving nature of AI, yet supervising adaptive, continuously learning models remains a complex task within traditionally static regulatory structures. The opacity of many advanced AI models, often described as operating within a "black box," further complicates efforts to interpret their decisions, posing challenges for transparency, trust, and ethical governance.

Collaboration and standardization between industry and academia are essential for advancing AI-driven drug discovery, though these partnerships must contend with barriers such as differing priorities, intellectual property issues, and information silos. Initiatives promoting data interoperability and traceability, such as those led by HL7 FHIR and CDISC, are vital for building reliable AI datasets and supporting rigorous regulatory review. Ensuring that these collaborative efforts uphold principles of equity is critical to expanding access to AI-enabled therapeutic advancements.

In conclusion, the responsible adoption of AI in pharmaceuticals demands robust governance, strong ethical standards, and international cooperation. Only through a comprehensive and coordinated approach can the sector fully realize AI's potential to deliver safe, effective, and accessible medicines.

References

1. AI Driven Drug Discovery: 5 Powerful Breakthroughs in 2025—Lifebit. Weblink: https://lifebit.ai/blog/ai-driven-drug-discovery/. Accessed June 2025.
2. How is AI used for drug repurposing in biopharma? Weblink: https://synapse.patsnap.com/article/how-is-ai-used-for-drug-repurposing-in-biopharma. Accessed June 2025.
3. Ethics and Governance of Artificial Intelligence for Healthcare. Weblink: https://iris.who.int/bitstream/handle/10665/341996/9789240029200-eng.pdf. Accessed June 2025.
4. Ethical considerations in AI-driven drug discovery. Weblink: https://prism.sustainability-directory.com/scenario/ethical-considerations-in-ai-driven-drug-discovery/. Accessed June 2025.

5. What are the limitations of using data anonymization techniques in conjunction with other AI-driven healthcare security measures? Weblink: https://massedcompute.com/faq-answers/?question=What+are+the+limitations+of+using+data+anonymization+techniques+in+conjunction+with+other+AI-driven+healthcare+security+measures?. Accessed June 2025.
6. Data anonymization: techniques, pros & cons, Weblink: https://www.syntho.ai/what-is-data-anonymization/. Accessed June 2025.
7. Venkatesaramani R, Malin BA, Vorobeychik Y. Re-identification of individuals in genomic datasets using public face images. Sci Adv. 2021;7(47):eabg3296.
8. Drakshpalli R. AI-driven threat detection in pharmaceutical R and D: mitigating cyber risks in drug discovery platforms. Glob J Eng Technol Adv. 2025;23(03):48–62.
9. Colombi C. AI data breaches in healthcare: protecting patient privacy & trust. 2025. Weblink: https://www.tonic.ai/blog/ai-data-breaches-in-healthcare. Accessed June 2025.
10. Navigate the FDA draft guidance on artificial intelligence (AI) and cybersecurity. Weblink: https://www.medcrypt.com/blog/navigate-the-fda-draft-guidance-on-artificial-intelligence-ai-and-cybersecurity. Accessed June 2025.
11. Hill T. Data privacy and protection in AI for precision medicine. 2023. Weblink: https://www.reprocell.com/blog/data-privacy-and-protection-in-ai-for-precision-medicine. Accessed June 2025.
12. Streamlining pharmacogenomics with data integration. Weblink: https://www.numberanalytics.com/blog/streamlining-pharmacogenomics-with-data-integration. Accessed June 2025.
13. Sharma S. Federated learning for privacy preserving AI: an IN-depth exploration. 2024. Weblink: https://roundtable.datascience.salon/federated-learning-for-privacy-preserving-ai-an-in-depth-exploration. Accessed June 2025.
14. How the FDA guidance on the use of AI will impact drug development. Weblink: https://www.pharmalex.com/thought-leadership/blogs/how-the-fda-guidance-on-the-use-of-ai-will-impact-drug-development/. Accessed July 2025.
15. https://www.fda.gov/regulatory-information/search-fda-guidance-documents/considerations-use-artificial-intelligence-support-regulatory-decision-making-drug-and-biological. Accessed July 2025.
16. Pradhan N. AI drug development: FDA releases draft guidance. 2025. Weblink: https://natlawreview.com/article/ai-drug-development-fda-releases-draft-guidance. Accessed July 2025.
17. Artificial intelligence for drug development. Weblink: https://www.fda.gov/about-fda/center-drug-evaluation-and-research-cder/artificial-intelligence-drug-development. Accessed July 2025.
18. European Medicines Agency. Reflection paper on the use of artificial intelligence (AI) in the medicinal product lifecycle. 2025. Weblink: https://www.ema.europa.eu/en/documents/scientific-guideline/reflection-paper-use-artificial-intelligence-ai-medicinal-product-lifecycle_en.pdf. Accessed July 2025.
19. EMA'S new work plan: leveraging data and AI to encourage innovation and research. Weblink: https://www.hoganlovells.com/en/publications/emas-new-work-plan-leveraging-data-and-ai-to-encourage-innovation-and-research. Accessed July 2025.
20. EFPIA position on the use of artificial intelligence in the medicinal product lifecycle. 2024. Weblink: https://efpia.eu/media/tzeavw1t/efpia-position-on-the-use-of-artificial-intelligence-in-the-medicinal-product-lifecycle.pdf. Accessed July 2025.
21. Ethics of artificial intelligence. Weblink: https://www.unesco.org/en/artificial-intelligence/recommendation-ethics. Accessed July 2025.
22. AI in drug development: FDA draft guidance addresses product lifecycle, risk. Weblink: https://www.raps.org/news-and-articles/news-articles/2025/1/ai-in-drug-development-fda-draft-guidance-addresse. Accessed July 2025.

23. Abulibdeh R, Celi LA, Sejdić E. The illusion of safety: a report to the FDA on AI healthcare product approvals. PLOS Digit Health. 2025;4(6):e0000866.
24. Use of fast healthcare interoperability resources (FHIR) in the generation of real world evidence (RWE). Weblink: https://www.cdisc.org/kb/articles/use-fast-healthcare-interoperability-resources-fhir-generation-real-world-evidence-rwe. Accessed July 2025.
25. EMA and HMA launch 2028 plan to use AI and real-world data in EU medicines regulation. Weblink: https://becarispublishing.com/digital-content/blog-post/ema-and-hma-launch-2028-plan-use-ai-and-real-world-data-eu-medicines-regulation. Accessed July 2025.
26. Pillai V. Enhancing transparency and understanding in AI decision-making processes. Iconic Res Eng J. 2024;8(1):168–72.
27. PAICON. WHO report explores the benefits and challenges of AI in pharmaceutical development. 2024. Weblink: https://paicon.com/news/ai-in-pharmaceutical-development/. Accessed July 2025.
28. Niazi SK. Regulatory perspectives for AI/ML implementation in pharmaceutical GMP environments. Pharmaceuticals. 2025;18(6):901.
29. Hulsen T. Explainable artificial intelligence (XAI): concepts and challenges in healthcare. Ai. 2023;4(3):652–66.
30. Grover V, Dogra M. Challenges and limitations of explainable AI in healthcare. In: Analyzing explainable AI in healthcare and the pharmaceutical industry. IGI Global Scientific Publishing; 2024. p. 72–85.
31. Taofeek A, Oluwaferanmi A, Hamzah F, Philp A, Liang B, John B. Intergrating multi-omics data using AI in Pharamacogenomics. 2025. Weblink: https://www.researchgate.net/publication/392082901_Integrating_Multi-Omics_Data_Using_AI_in_Pharmacogenomics. Accessed July 2025.
32. Bagad S. Beyond expectations: transforming life sciences through AI-drive multi-omics integration. 2025. Weblink: https://www.bc-la.org/consulting-2/beyond-expectations%3A-transforming-life-sciences-through-ai-driven-multi-omics-integration-. Accessed July 2025.
33. Verma V, Manocha N, Patel R, Agrawal G, Chhabra G. Accelerating drug discovery and development through artificial intelligence: challenges and opportunities. Int J Pharm Sci. 2025;3(6):3160.
34. Dermawan D, Alotaiq N. From lab to clinic: how artificial intelligence (AI) is reshaping drug discovery timelines and industry outcomes. Pharmaceuticals. 2025;18(7):981.
35. Artificial intelligence in pharmaceuticals and biotechnology: current trends and innovations. Weblink: https://www.coherentsolutions.com/insights/artificial-intelligence-in-pharmaceuticals-and-biotechnology-current-trends-and-innovations. Accessed July 2025.
36. AI in the pharmaceutical industry. Weblink: https://digitaldefynd.com/IQ/ai-in-pharmaceutical-industry/. Accessed July 2025.
37. Loveth RG. Emerging technologies in AI-driven biotech innovations. 2025.
38. FDA AI Guidance—A new era for biotech, diagnostics and regulatory compliance. 2025. Weblink: https://www.duanemorris.com/alerts/fda_ai_guidance_new_era_biotech_diagnostics_regulatory_compliance_0225.html. Accessed July 2025.
39. Palaniappan K, Lin EYT, Vogel S. Global regulatory frameworks for the use of artificial intelligence (AI) in the healthcare services sector. Healthcare. 2024;12(5):562.
40. HL7 international publishes new report from HL7 outlines how AI-supported by standards and interoperability—can tackle healthcare fraud. Weblink: https://blog.hl7.org/hl7-new-report-from-hl7-outlines-how-ai-supported-by-standards-and-interoperability-can-tackle-healthcare-fraud. Accessed July 2025.

Future Trends and Innovations in AI-Driven Drug Development

7

The pharmaceutical industry, traditionally characterized by lengthy timelines and high costs, is undergoing a profound transformation driven by artificial intelligence (AI). AI's current impact is already evident in accelerating drug discovery, optimizing clinical trials, and enhancing manufacturing processes. This chapter delves into the cutting-edge trends and innovations poised to further reshape the future of AI-driven drug development, exploring the synergistic integration of AI with robotics, its pivotal role in decentralized clinical trials, the disruptive potential of quantum computing and next-generation AI models, and a strategic roadmap addressing critical ethical, regulatory, and collaborative imperatives.

7.1 Integration of AI with Robotics and Automation

The convergence of AI and robotics is fundamentally reshaping the drug development lifecycle, moving beyond theoretical promise to tangible operational impacts across discovery, preclinical research, manufacturing, and supply chain.

7.1.1 AI-Powered Automation in Drug Discovery and Preclinical Research

The fusion of AI and robotics is transforming drug discovery and preclinical research, especially the design, make, test, analyze (DMTA) cycle. AI excels at molecular property prediction, virtual screening, and de novo molecule design, while robotics automates synthesis and repetitive tasks, enabling scientists to quickly explore chemical spaces and refine experiments. Notable advancements include generative AI (GenAI) for early-stage

K. Shaikh et al., *Artificial Intelligence in Drug Discovery and Development*,
Synthesis Lectures on Engineering, Science, and Technology,
https://doi.org/10.1007/978-3-032-10277-5_7

design, AlphaFold's accurate 3D protein structure prediction, and platforms like Iktos Robotics and Atomwise's AtomNet, which offer end-to-end AI-driven automation to screen and design millions of compounds efficiently and identify novel drug candidates [1–5].

High-throughput screening (HTS) is revolutionized by AI, leveraging machine learning, deep learning, and graph neural networks to identify hits more rapidly and reliably [6]. AI's ability to monitor assays in real time, optimize conditions, and reduce errors allows drug development timelines to shrink from over a decade to as little as 3–6 years, cutting costs up to 70% [2, 6]. This shift from trial-and-error to rational, AI-driven design improves success rates in clinical trials and could save the industry up to $410 billion annually by 2025 [7]; closed-loop discovery systems now allow AI to guide robots from design to testing, iteratively refining compounds and streamlining the entire process [1, 8, 9].

7.1.2 AI in Automated Drug Manufacturing and Supply Chain Optimization

AI and machine learning are dramatically improving efficiency and reliability in drug manufacturing, with predictive maintenance increasing uptime by 15–20% [7] and digital twins enabling real-time process optimization [10]. Companies like Pfizer have leveraged generative AI to boost manufacturing throughput by 20%, optimizing vaccine production and dramatically shortening timelines for critical drugs such as the COVID-19 vaccine to just 269 days [10]. In the supply chain, AI-driven predictive analytics and IoT sensors enable accurate demand forecasting, inventory management, and real-time tracking, safeguarding cold chain products and combating counterfeit drugs with blockchain-enabled traceability [11–13].

AI transitions pharmaceutical operations from reactive to proactive, anticipating equipment failures, identifying supply bottlenecks, and enhancing resilience across the value chain [7, 12, 14]. However, widespread adoption brings challenges like high initial costs, integration with legacy systems, regulatory hurdles, and workforce adaptation [15]. Addressing these issues requires investment not only in technology but also in training and upskilling staff to work with AI systems, ensuring effective management and a collaborative human-AI ecosystem [15].

7.2 AI in Decentralized and Digital Trials

AI has transformed clinical transformed clinical trials by enabling adaptive "smart" protocols that respond to real-time data, improving flexibility and efficiency in study design [16]. Notably, AI and machine learning streamline patient recruitment, a process that historically accounts for about 30% of total trial timelines [11]. Tools like IBM Watson for clinical trial matching at the Mayo clinic have significantly increased trail matching rates and reduced eligibility screening times [16], while Deep AI rapidly identified qualified participants from millions of records, vastly outpacing traditional methods [16]. "Precision recruitment" using advanced analytics allows studies to efficiently target individuals most likely to benefit, as demonstrated by companies like Icarus Therapeutics applying AI to match patients remotely and within specific regions [16].

AI also enhances trial design and monitoring, predicting and addressing operational challenges early [17]. Advanced analytics continually track recruitment, adherence, and safety signals, applying machine learning to forecast risks such as underperforming sites or increased dropouts [17]. This proactive monitoring supports timely interventions for smoother progress. Additionally, refining inclusion criteria with AI shortens trial durations by 10% and is estimated to save the industry $25 billion annually while also improving population representation [7]. A recent development in the field is the use of digital twins, virtual patient models combining real-world data and simulations to predict treatment responses and optimize dosages [16]. Digital twins can simulate full trial outcomes before enrolling any participants, reducing time and potential costs. Companies like Unlearn AI employ digital twin technology (TwinRCTs) to decrease required enrollment in late-stage studies while maintaining statistical power [16].

Overall, the evolution of clinical trials driven by AI enhances accessibility and adaptability. Decentralized trials, supported by AI, allow broader patient participation by overcoming geographical barriers, increasing diversity, and improving relevance of findings [7]. Real-time data analysis enables continuous protocol optimization, making trials more efficient and reflective of real-world conditions [8]. Together, these advancements improve recruitment, retention, and, ultimately, patient outcomes and research robustness.

7.3 Quantum Computing and Next-Gen AI Models

The future of AI-driven drug development will be profoundly shaped by the emergence of quantum computing and advances in next-generation AI models, pushing the boundaries of computational power and molecular understanding.

7.3.1 Quantum Computing's Impact on Drug Discovery

Quantum computing (QC) is a transformative technology poised to revolutionize drug discovery and healthcare by overcoming the computational limitations inherent in classical methods and even traditional AI [18]. While classical AI excels in pattern recognition and predictive modeling, it encounters significant challenges when simulating highly complex molecular interactions, protein folding, and atomic-level quantum states due to its reliance on approximations and extensive computational resources [18]. QC offers a fundamentally different approach by leveraging qubits and quantum mechanical principles like superposition and entanglement to simulate nature at its most basic level, modeling the behavior of molecules, atoms, and electrons with much higher fidelity [18].

One of the most promising applications of QC is in quantum molecular simulations. Quantum algorithms like the variational quantum eigensolver (VQE) and quantum phase estimation (QPE) are used to calculate molecular energy states and binding affinities more precisely than classical methods [18]. This capability can accelerate the process of studying protein-ligand binding, a crucial step in drug development, by up to 100 million times faster than classical supercomputers [19]. In drug optimization and design, quantum annealing, a unique quantum computing approach, is particularly effective for solving optimization problems. It finds the lowest energy state of a system, enabling the exploration of vast energy landscapes of molecular configurations to maximize desired properties [20]. Furthermore, quantum machine learning (QML) merges QC with AI, enhancing capabilities in virtual screening, molecular classification, and compound clustering [18]. QML models can encode molecular features into quantum states, accelerating model training and inference, especially in high-dimensional datasets [18].

The integration of quantum computing represents a profound acceleration of fundamental understanding in drug discovery. QC does not merely speed up existing computational processes; it enables a fundamentally different approach to modeling nature at its most basic level [21]. This allows for a deeper and more accurate understanding of biochemistry and complex molecular behavior, moving beyond approximations that limit classical AI. This enhanced comprehension of underlying biological mechanisms is crucial for developing truly novel therapeutic strategies, rather than just optimizing existing ones. By providing insights into quantum mechanical processes, QC facilitates the design of drugs with unprecedented precision and efficacy, promising breakthroughs that were previously computationally intractable.

7.3.2 Next-Generation AI Models (Beyond Traditional ML/DL)

Beyond quantum computing, the evolution of AI models themselves is driving significant innovation. Foundation models (FMs) emerge as inherently versatile tools, pretrained on a wide range of data to cater to multiple downstream tasks without requiring reinitialization of parameters [22]. In bioinformatics, FMs primarily focus on core biological problems, including biological sequence analysis, biological structure construction, and biological function prediction, learning from both annotated and unannotated biological datasets [22]. They are capable of learning accurate representations of intricate biological datasets, tailoring large language models (LLMs) for biological problems through fine-tuning processes [22].

Protein foundation models, such as AlphaFold 3, ESM-3, and Proteína, are transforming protein research by learning the rules of folding, function, and evolution within a single, reusable neural network [23]. These models unify various protein-related tasks including fold prediction, mutational scanning, docking, and de novo design into one promotable engine, potentially turning weeks of lab work or code into minutes of inference [23]. This promises to reshape protein R&D into a software-first workflow, with future models moving beyond folding to full-scale fabrication, designing multi-chain complexes, metabolic pathways, and even adaptive biomaterials on demand [23].

Generative AI, a subset of these next-generation models, continues to play a pivotal role in creating brand-new molecular structures and optimizing their chemical properties, moving drug discovery from screening existing compounds to intelligently designing novel ones [3]. These next-generation AI models represent a significant paradigm shift in molecular design and discovery. Instead of relying solely on predictive analytics applied to existing datasets, these models possess generative capabilities that allow them to create novel biological entities and molecular structures from scratch [1]. This enables the exploration of previously uncharted chemical spaces and the design of complex multi-chain complexes or metabolic pathways, which were beyond the scope of traditional methods or even earlier AI algorithms. This generative capacity promises to unlock entirely new avenues for therapeutic development, leading to breakthroughs that were previously unimaginable and fundamentally reshaping the drug discovery process.

7.3.3 Challenges and Limitations

Despite their immense potential, both quantum computing and next-generation AI models face significant challenges that must be addressed for widespread adoption in drug development. For quantum computing, key challenges include hardware noise, a limited number of stable qubits, and high error rates [18]. Maintaining qubit coherence, the ability of qubits to retain their quantum states becomes increasingly difficult as systems scale, as they are extremely sensitive to environmental noise [24]. Interconnect and control challenges also grow with system size, creating bottlenecks and calibration hurdles [24]. Furthermore, current quantum algorithms often assume ideal qubits, but real-world systems require accounting for noise, connectivity constraints, and hardware-specific quirks, complicating software and algorithm development [24]. While innovations are reducing qubit requirements and improving error correction, these remain active areas of research [25].

Next-generation AI models also present limitations. Data quality remains paramount, as these sophisticated algorithms require high-quality data to learn and make accurate predictions [21]. A significant challenge is the interpretability of these complex models, often referred to as their "black box" nature [26]. Understanding the basis for their predictions is crucial for regulatory acceptance, trust, and identifying potential biases [26]. Robust validation frameworks are essential to ensure the reliability and generalizability of these models in real-world clinical settings [27].

Bridging the gap from theoretical promise to practical application for these advanced technologies requires concerted effort. While these technologies demonstrate impressive technical benchmarks in controlled environments, their practical implementation faces significant hurdles related to operational variability, data heterogeneity, and integration with existing workflows [27]. This indicates that success depends not solely on algorithmic innovation but also on substantial advancements in hardware, data infrastructure, and the development of adaptable regulatory frameworks [27]. The focus must shift from merely achieving high performance in idealized settings to ensuring seamless integration, real-world reliability, and clinical utility.

7.4 Roadmap for Future Drug Development Strategies

The rapid evolution of AI in drug development requires a strategic approach that considers technology, ethics, regulation, and collaboration.

7.4.1 Ethical and Regulatory Frameworks

AI-driven drug discovery relies on large, sensitive datasets, raising privacy and security concerns, such as data re-identification, model poisoning, and adversarial attacks [28–30]. Solutions include encryption, strong anonymization, and emerging technologies like homomorphic encryption [31], though these can impact data quality [32]. Bias in training data can perpetuate health disparities [28, 33]. To address this, diverse data and bias-mitigation techniques are essential. Explainability (XAI) is increasingly required by regulators, though it can be challenging to balance with accuracy [26, 34, 35]. Regulatory bodies (FDA, EMA) are adapting by issuing new guidance and emphasizing data transparency, lifecycle maintenance, and early engagement [36–38]. The regulatory landscape must remain dynamic to ensure safety, privacy, and equitable access [26, 28, 36, 38].

7.4.2 Collaborative Ecosystems and Data Standardization

Effective AI in drug development depends on partnerships and standardizing data formats. Industry-academic collaboration speeds innovation but faces obstacles like IP rights and data silos [7]. Standardization initiatives such as FHIR and CDISC are vital for harmonizing and integrating diverse datasets [39–42], supporting scalable AI and precision medicine. Without standardization, the potential of AI to produce effective therapies remains limited [40, 43].

7.4.3 Societal Impact and Equitable Access

AI can address rare diseases by shortening diagnostic time and improving research despite limited data [44–46]. It also advances personalized medicine through genomic data analysis and tailored therapies [47–49]. However, there is a risk that AI benefits will be concentrated in wealthier regions [28]. To prevent widening health inequities, proactive measures for equitable access, diverse data representation, and global collaboration are needed [28]. The aim is to ensure AI advances health for all communities worldwide.

In summary, the integration of artificial intelligence into drug development is rapidly transforming the pharmaceutical landscape. The convergence of AI with robotics and automation is streamlining the DMTA cycle, enabling more efficient, precise, and personalized approaches to drug discovery. These advancements are accelerating timelines, reducing costs, and enhancing the quality of drug candidates while also demanding new skills and fostering collaboration between humans and intelligent systems. Moreover, AI is revolutionizing clinical trials through decentralized, patient-centric models, leveraging smart protocols, digital twins, and AI-driven recruitment to make research more accessible and responsive to diverse populations.

Looking toward the future, breakthroughs in quantum computing and next-generation AI models promise to unlock deeper understanding of molecular biology and usher in a new era of therapeutic innovation. However, to fully realize the transformative potential of these technologies, the industry must navigate complex ethical and regulatory challenges, ensuring robust safeguards around data privacy, fairness, and equitable access. By prioritizing ethical frameworks, investing in adaptable infrastructure, and fostering global partnerships, the pharmaceutical sector can harness the power of AI to deliver safer, more effective medicines for all, and rise to meet the needs of both common and rare disease communities alike.

References

1. The future of generative AI and automation in drug discovery. Weblink: https://www.iptonline.com/articles/the-future-of-generative-ai-and-automation-in-drug-discovery. Accessed July 2025.
2. Bioinformatics meets AI: a match made in drug discovery heaven. Weblink: https://lifebit.ai/blog/ai-driven-drug-discovery/. Accessed July 2025.
3. Wan Z, Sun X, Li Y, Chu T, Hao X, Cao Y, Zhang P. Applications of artificial intelligence in drug repurposing. Adv Sci. 2025;12(14):2411325.
4. AI in the pharmaceutical industry [5 success stories] [2025]. Weblink: https://digitaldefynd.com/IQ/ai-in-pharmaceutical-industry/. Accessed July 2025.
5. 12 AI drug discovery companies you should know about. Weblink: https://www.labiotech.eu/best-biotech/ai-drug-discovery-companies/. Accessed: July 2025.
6. What role does AI play in high-throughput screening for drug discovery? Weblink: https://synapse.patsnap.com/article/what-role-does-ai-play-in-high-throughput-screening-for-drug-discovery. Accessed July 2025.
7. Inside the cross-sector collaborations driving AI in biotech. Weblink: https://www.azorobotics.com/Article.aspx?ArticleID=760. Accessed July 2025.
8. Tomar P, Goel F, Pal A, Garg VK. The future of drug development: leveraging AI for faster and safer innovation. J Adv Sci Res. 2025;16(04):5–11.

9. Why drug discovery needs robots and artificial intelligence. Weblink: https://www.news-medical.net/health/Why-Drug-Discovery-Needs-Robots-and-Artificial-Intelligence.aspx. Accessed July 2025.
10. How AI drug manufacturing is changing the game. Weblink: https://healthtechmagazine.net/article/2025/02/ai-in-drug-manufacturing-perfcon. Accessed July 2025.
11. How AI is reshaping pharma: use cases, challenges. Weblink: https://whatfix.com/blog/ai-in-pharma/. Accessed July 2025.
12. AI and automation in pharma supply chain management. Weblink: https://www.eawlogistics.com/ai-and-automation-in-pharma-supply-chain-management/. Accessed July 2025.
13. The impact of AI & automation in pharmaceutical supply chains. Weblink: https://www.pharmasolutions-int.com/the-impact-of-ai-automation-in-pharmaceutical-supply-chains/. Accessed July 2025.
14. Saini JPS, Thakur A, Yadav D. AI driven innovations in pharmaceuticals: optimizing drug discovery and industry operations. RSC Pharmaceutics. 2025;2:437.
15. The role of robotics and AI in pharmaceutical automation. Weblink: https://www.pharmafocuseurope.com/articles/the-role-of-robotics-and-ai-in-pharmaceutical-automation. Accessed July 2025.
16. The evolution of decentralized clinical trials: blending innovation and regulation in the digital age. Weblink: https://globalforum.diaglobal.org/issue/october-2024/the-evolution-of-decentralized-clinical-trials-blending-innovation-and-regulation-in-the-digital-age/. Accessed July 2025.
17. How is AI addressing patient recruitment challenges and speeding up clinical trial timelines? Weblink: https://trialx.com/how-is-ai-addressing-patient-recruitment-challenges-and-speeding-up-clinical-trial-timelines/. Accessed July 2025.
18. Palle S. Advancing drug discovery with quantum computing breaking artificial intelligence barriers. 2025. Weblink: https://nhsjs.com/2025/advancing-drug-discovery-with-quantum-computing-breaking-artificial-intelligence-barriers/. Accessed July 2025.
19. Quantum computing in drug discovery: quantum molecular simulations. Weblink: https://quantumzeitgeist.com/quantum-computing-in-drug-discovery-quantum-molecular-simulations/. Accessed July 2025.
20. Bishwas AK, Pitchai A, Som A. Molecular unfolding formulation with enhanced quantum annealing approach. 2024. arXiv preprint arXiv:2403.00507.
21. Ferreira FJ, Carneiro AS. AI-driven drug discovery: a comprehensive review. ACS Omega. 2025;10:23889.
22. Quantum computing in pharma and chemistry. Weblink: https://www.classiq.io/industries/industries-chemistry-pharma. Accessed July 2025.
23. Biomolecular foundation models for discovery in life science. Weblink: https://www.nvidia.com/en-us/use-cases/biomolecular-foundation-models-for-discovery-in-life-science/. Accessed July 2025.
24. What are the challenges of scaling up qubit systems? Weblink: https://milvus.io/ai-quick-reference/what-are-the-challenges-of-scaling-up-qubit-systems. Accessed July 2025.
25. Quantiuum overcomes last major hurdle to deliver scalable universal fault-tolerant quantum computers by 2029. Weblink: https://www.quantinuum.com/blog/quantinuum-overcomes-last-major-hurdle-to-deliver-scalable-universal-fault-tolerant-quantum-computers-by-2029. Accessed July 2025.
26. Niazi SK. Regulatory perspectives for AI/ML implementation in pharmaceutical GMP environments. Pharmaceuticals. 2025;18(6):901.
27. AI in drug development: clinical validation and regulatory innovation are dual imperatives. Weblink: https://globalforum.diaglobal.org/issue/june-2025/ai-in-drug-development-clinical-validation-and-regulatory-innovation-are-dual-imperatives/. Accessed July 2025.

28. Ethical considerations in AI-driven drug discovery. Weblink: https://prism.sustainability-directory.com/scenario/ethical-considerations-in-ai-driven-drug-discovery/. Accessed July 2025.
29. Venkatesaramani R, Malin BA, Vorobeychik Y. Re-identification of individuals in genomic datasets using public face images. Sci Adv. 2021;7(47):eabg3296.
30. Drakshpalli R. AI-driven threat detection in pharmaceutical R and D: mitigating cyber risks in drug discovery platforms. Glob J Eng Technol Adv. 2025;23(3):048–62.
31. The future of fully homomorphic encryption (FHE). Weblink: https://www.iotinsider.com/industries/security/the-future-of-fully-homomorphic-encryption-fhe/. Accessed July 2025.
32. Limitations of data anonymization techniques in AI-driven healthcare security. Weblink: https://massedcompute.com/faq-answers/?question=What+are+the+limitations+of+using+data+anonymization+techniques+in+conjunction+with+other+AI-driven+healthcare+security+measures? Accessed July 2025.
33. Health and AI: advancing responsible and ethical AI for all communities. Weblink: https://www.brookings.edu/articles/health-and-ai-advancing-responsible-and-ethical-ai-for-all-communities/. Accessed July 2025.
34. Ethics and governance of artificial intelligence for health. Weblink: https://iris.who.int/bitstream/handle/10665/341996/9789240029200-eng.pdf. Accessed April 2025.
35. Pillai V. Enhancing transparency and understanding in AI decision-making processes. Iconic Res Eng J. 2024;8(1):168–72.
36. How the FDA guidance on the use of AI will impact drug development. Weblink: https://www.pharmalex.com/thought-leadership/blogs/how-the-fda-guidance-on-the-use-of-ai-will-impact-drug-development/. Accessed June 2025.
37. EMA and HMA launch 2028 plan to use AI and real-world data in EU medicines regulation. Weblink: https://becarispublishing.com/digital-content/blog-post/ema-and-hma-launch-2028-plan-use-ai-and-real-world-data-eu-medicines-regulation. Accessed June 2025.
38. Reflection paper on the use of Artificial Intelligence (AI) in the medicinal product lifecycle. Weblink: https://www.ema.europa.eu/en/documents/scientific-guideline/reflection-paper-use-artificial-intelligence-ai-medicinal-product-lifecycle_en.pdf. Accessed June 2025.
39. Taofeek A, Oluwaferanmi A, Hamzah F, Philp A, Johnson B, Liang W, John B. Integrating multi-omics data using AI in pharmacogenomics. 2025. Weblink: https://www.researchgate.net/publication/392082901_Integrating_Multi-Omics_Data_Using_AI_in_Pharmacogenomics. Accessed June 2025.
40. Streamlining pharmacogenomics with data integration. Weblink: https://www.numberanalytics.com/blog/streamlining-pharmacogenomics-with-data-integration. Accessed June 2025.
41. HL7 international publishes new report from HL7 outlines How AI-Supported by standards and interoperability-can tackle healthcare fraud. Weblink: https://blog.hl7.org/hl7-new-report-from-hl7-outlines-how-ai-supported-by-standards-and-interoperability-can-tackle-healthcare-fraud. Accessed June 2025.
42. Zopf R, Abolafia J, Reddy B. Use of fast healthcare interoperability resources (FHIR) in the generation of real world evidence (RWE). In: Proceedings of PhUSE. Edinburgh, UK.; 2017.
43. How is AI used for drug repurposing in biopharma? Weblink: https://synapse.patsnap.com/article/how-is-ai-used-for-drug-repurposing-in-biopharma. Accessed June 2025.
44. Williamson K. How AI is addressing drug development challenges in rare diseases. 2025. Weblink: https://www.pharmafocuseurope.com/articles/how-ai-is-addressing-drug-development-challenges-in-rare-diseases. Accessed June 2025.
45. The diagnostic odyssey: The search for answers for rare diseases. Weblink: https://medicover-genetics.com/the-diagnostic-odyssey-the-search-for-answers-for-rare-diseases/. Accessed June 2025.

46. AI drug repurposing helps find medicine for rare disease. Weblink: https://www.technologynetworks.com/drug-discovery/news/ai-drug-repurposing-helps-find-medicine-for-rare-disease-395863. Accessed June 2025.
47. Nelson J. AI in personalized medicine: tailoring treatments based on patient data. 2025
48. AI in pharmacogenomics: a comprehensive guide. Weblink: https://www.numberanalytics.com/blog/ai-in-pharmacogenomics-guide. Accessed June 2025.
49. The future of drug design: emerging trends. Weblink: https://www.numberanalytics.com/blog/future-drug-design-emerging-trends. Accessed June 2025.

Index

K. Shaikh et al., *Artificial Intelligence in Drug Discovery and Development*, Synthesis Lectures on Engineering, Science, and Technology, https://doi.org/10.1007/978-3-032-10277-5

MIX
Papier aus verantwortungsvollen Quellen
Paper from responsible sources
FSC® C105338

If you have any concerns about our products,
you can contact us on
ProductSafety@springernature.com

In case Publisher is established outside the EU,
the EU authorized representative is:
Springer Nature Customer Service Center GmbH
Europaplatz 3, 69115 Heidelberg, Germany

Printed by Libri Plureos GmbH
in Hamburg, Germany